DEALING ADDICTION

DEALING ADDICTION

HOW THE CANADIAN GOVERNMENT DERAILED ADDICTION RECOVERY

KAREN JAMES

atmosphere press

Published by Atmosphere Press

Cover design by Matthew Fielder

Arrow icon sourced from Vecteezy.com

Atmospherepress.com

Dedicated to

Mildred James (McGrath)

1915–1976

To all of you who died unnecessarily

Foreword

I have known Karen James for nearly 20 years, and I have never met anyone who has given so much of her time and of herself to others. I've seen, up close and personal, how years of working within a system that lacks both adequate resources and, sometimes, the courage to question itself have often taken a toll on her mental and physical health. Yet, she gets up and tries again. And again.

Dealing Addiction is Karen's story, a point of view – intensely personal, unflinchingly honest, and unapologetic.

She challenges us to confront uncomfortable truths. Her insights into harm reduction, systemic neglect, and the collateral damage inflicted on families and communities should lead us to question many of our assumptions. She also does not shy away from exploring the broader implications of addiction, asking hard questions about its economic, social, and psychological costs. At the same time, she places a vital emphasis on recovery – what it requires, what it promises, and why it matters. Because it's where hope lies.

Some readers will take issue with her views; others will find in them a voice they've been waiting to hear. But this book is not an invitation to agree or disagree. It is a call to listen and to dialogue.

MJ.

Contents

Introduction

Addiction is a significant issue that dominates the news and delivers very extreme images of what often looks like scenes from the walking dead. How did it get this bad because it has become worse? The common response is usually, it's the drugs they use these days. They've gotten worse, so the situation is out of hand. I believe that there's more to why it's gotten so bad, and it's not just the drugs, it's our response to the problem.

The response to addiction has a history that dates back to a time when we saw addicts as morally degenerate and in need of being straightened out, through many different revisions of this attitude, as we struggled to understand just what was going on that caused some people to become addicted while others did not. Unfortunately, this was not just a genuine search for answers because it was also influenced by politics and funding. This affected those who did the job of working with people with addictions and what kind of help they would be entitled to.

Funding shaped a lot of what was done or not done, including who got help and who did not. When I first entered the addiction world in 1992, if you weren't a sure bet, they dumped you because statistics ensured funding, so if you weren't going to make it, it was better to kick you out before you were counted. One has to remember this was at a time when those with addiction weren't really liked very much. The pendulum would swing back and forth over the years.

This is the problem with addiction. It has never been approached as the problem that it is with all the issues it brings with it. We cannot view it in isolation. It does not just affect the addicted person but has a much broader impact, and when one does not factor in that broader impact, we fail to get it right every time. We have to understand its biology and neuropsychology. We have to understand what in our society is contributing to it. We have to look at the effect it is having on families and, in particular, children. We need to look at the effect it is having on neighborhoods and small businesses. How is it impacting hospitals and crime rates? How much is it contributing to increases in violence? What about the transmission of diseases such as COVID? When we take all of this into account, we cannot afford to not treat addiction because the damage of not treating it is far too great.

Despite everything I have just mentioned, Canada, in all of its infinite wisdom, has decided that the best approach to addiction is to just sustain it under the guise of Harm Reduction. It takes this position like it is the true compassionate advocate of those with substance use disorders, stating that it is offering life-saving measures to allow these people to live their lives the way they want to live their lives. They will bring them back from an overdose. This does nothing to describe the quality of the lives these people are living but it somehow tries to equate itself with the idea of dignity.

***

Harm Reduction as an approach has meant different things at different times. Originally, it meant approaches that sought to reduce the harm caused by using substances. This would include things like clean needles, clean supplies, needle dispensaries, needle discard boxes, and anything else that would help people so that the risk of infection and disease would be reduced. It expanded to the provision of places where people could inject their drugs so the risk of overdose could be reduced and the provision of Narcan for overdoses. There were places that could check drugs for the presence of fentanyl or other problem substances. Eventually, it included the decriminalization of smaller quantities of substances and then the provision of prescription drugs that equated to the commonly used drugs, thereby providing a safe supply. This has moved the attitude towards drug use to one of choice where it is acceptable for people to choose to be substance users, and this is viewed and supported as an acceptable way of life.

If you ask addicted people what they want, they will opt for the right to use substances. You can engage addicted people in services, and this is done by offering them things that they might want, like food, clothing, housing and drugs. This looks like a reasonable and decent thing to do, except that addicted people use the things they get to sell to get money to buy illegal drugs. In essence, you create a second economy for them. The drugs that are given to addicted people are used by them along with the street drugs they continue to buy and use, or they are sold for street drugs. Providing drugs does not stop the purchase and use of street drugs, because you will never be willing to provide enough drugs that the addicted person wants. That amount is an unlimited supply.

The idea that people should have the right to use substances, despite the overwhelmingly negative effects their using drugs and alcohol has on other people, is questionable. The reason why society has not been sympathetic to people with addiction is precisely because their using drugs has broader effects. Neighborhoods have had to deal with actively using people on their streets who behave in extremely negative ways and who affect the quality of their lives. People under the influence do not behave well. People under the influence don't take other people into account. People who are using require money to purchase their drugs, whether legal or illegal.

When a person's use becomes chronic, they are often unable to participate meaningfully in society. They are often the financial recipients of social services because any money they have is diverted to pay for their drugs, and chronic use interferes with one's ability to work. Currently the focus is on giving them whatever they need to continue in their current lifestyle. Food banks provide them with food, housing first seeks to make sure they get housing and donations supply clothing. Startup programs provide them with furniture and household items. Many qualify for ODSP, which gives them access to several other supplementary items. They get money for a bus pass and a special dietary allowance if they can find a way to qualify. Most of them know how to work the system and get more than what they need, which then allows them to have extra money by supplying them with an inventory of items they can sell.

As their use gets more and more out of hand, illegal activities become necessary. They must steal to pay for their use. No one seems at all concerned about the many businesses that must absorb the costs that people using drugs take on them through theft. Alcoholics resort to stealing alcohol in order to meet their needs. Pharmacies have also been objects of break-ins and thefts. Coin-operated washers and dryers are often targeted as well, and that also includes people breaking into your apartment building and breaking your washer or dryer while removing the coins. Leaving people with no washer or dryer and forcing them to resort to paying three or four times as much to wash their clothes at a public coin wash.

These are some of the reasons why it's hard for many people to be sympathetic to people with addictions. A lot of the helping hand that has been offered to people with addictions has set up a dependency and an attitude and expectation that they should be given whatever they need. So rather than encouraging people to become meaningful members of society, we have trained them to become leeches upon society. They go from one service to another, taking everything they can get. We bribe them to come to our services, thinking we can somehow have some meaningful effect on them when all they come for is what they can get from us. I have seen addicted people fighting over what is offered freely to them and taking as much as they can carry, knowing that they intend to sell these items to make money to buy their drugs. What are we teaching them here?

If we look back on the notion of choice, then the question becomes, when one person's choices rob others of their quality of life, should that be acceptable? Knowing that addiction is not a choice, why are we not putting more money into the treatment of addiction instead of finding ways to sustain it? My argument is that the reason is that somebody is making enough money from it to make it become an issue of choice. My complaint is simple. Why are my rights worth less than the rights of actively using people since I live in one of the neighborhoods that house many active addicts? I live there because I work in the addiction field, and the stigma of addiction attaches to me, so I am not paid a salary that allows me the luxury of living in a higher income area.

My quality of life is affected daily as I have to walk through people hanging around on the streets, yelling and screaming profanities at each other. I have been assaulted by a person for simply saying hello to them. I cannot open my window on summer nights because the yelling and the partying goes on to the early hours of the morning, and I must get up early to go to work. I have also had to walk through an array of police cars parked all around the building where I live because some violent incident has taken place. Two different houses were the subjects of arson over a one-month period. No children play on the streets where I live. People scream out their offers of a blow job for money. One night six shots rang out right behind my bedroom window that left me paralyzed with fear. No sirens responded and no police came. Just another night in my neighborhood. These are a few of the kinds of experiences that people in these neighborhoods face.

I spoke to a man at a nearby convenience store and asked him how he finds running a business in this area. He said that women frequently come into his store and take what they want. If he challenges them, they simply put the item down the front of their pants and tell him to take it back. He said some women have offered to give him a blow job in exchange for taking what they want from his store. He says it is pointless to call the police because this does not change or resolve the problem. This is a regular occurrence for him.

Mix this in with people who are barely living a human existence, and yet somehow, we think that this is OK. Family members who have lost their loved ones to this unholy mess cannot retrieve them from the streets and just wait for the call that tells them they have died. Kids growing up with Dr. Jekyll and Mr. Hyde for a parent and can never trust who they are coming home to after school. Addiction can be treated, and people can recover. We know that. There's no need for what is going on in this country, so the question remains why we are not doing it.

***

I wanted to give some context to the story I want to tell. Too often the issue of addiction is not presented in its entirety. Either one side or another presents their story, but we never get the complete story. It depends on the current political position and whose voice gets heard the loudest. The pendulum swings back and forth and back and forth, and nothing ever gets resolved in a way that takes all parties into account. I am a recovered drug and alcohol addict. I am active in the recovering community. I grew up in an addicted home that resulted in the loss of both my parents. I worked in an addicted workplace for a substantial part of my early adulthood. I have worked in the field of addiction for over twenty-seven years. I have lived in an actively addiction-riddled neighborhood for over twenty years.

PART ONE:

GROWING UP IN ADDICTION

I was born into addiction; it was as normal as breathing. My mother's family was an Irish Catholic family that christened everything with alcohol. The kitchen table was forever covered with an assortment of bottles of booze. Every night was predictable if alcohol was on the table. Sooner or later a fight would ensue and then the despair would flow freely. Alcohol equaled anger and depression, as predictable as the reality that morning followed night. I kind of realized it was connected to the alcohol, but it was normal, so what else could you think? I remember I once believed that I would never drink because I was so tired of all the endless fighting that erupted after the family partook. It would only take one time to set my addiction in motion.

My mother's alcohol use released her anger and often she saw me as the cause of all her problems. The last child born into a disintegrating marriage; she told me she needed me as much as she needed two heads.

My father was both an alcoholic and a criminal, so he never added up to much as a father or a husband. My mother met him when they were both working for Producer's Dairy and they both liked to party. Their coworkers made a bet that their relationship would never last, so they got married to prove them wrong. He was fourteen years younger than she was and nowhere near the point of settling down to raise a family. He exited early from the family, running from charges that would have landed him in prison. He left with the woman who lived upstairs. He was the two things my mother hated the most: a liar and a thief. This left my mother as a single parent of three children.

When he was in our lives all he did was steal her money so he could go out drinking. That's what most of the fights between them were about. She needed money to take care of their kids, and he needed money to go out and drink. Over the years after he left, she would tell us many stories about him that would reveal how out of control he was. He was often arrested for being drunk and disorderly, and he forever fought with the police.

In one story she told, he had gotten drunk in a small town that was celebrating the town's birthday, and they had chosen to just let him sleep it off in the sheriff's office. He found a gun in a drawer and ended up shooting the end of his baby finger off. He called my mother to tell her he was bleeding to death, and she said good and slammed the phone down. When I met him as an adult it was the first thing I looked for and, sure enough, he was missing the end of his baby finger.

It was the early sixties, which was a time when women did not receive equal wages, so even though she would work twenty-five years as a lab technician in a dairy, she would never make enough to rise above her despair. We grew up in poverty and alcohol became the only escape that my mother could find. People often criticize the poor for spending money on booze, but when the little that you have won't make a difference, alcohol becomes the only antidote for despair, all-be-it a poor one at that. Drunkenness brought out her rage, her anger, her depression, and her bitterness. Home became a combat zone. The same bitter fights would be fought repeatedly.

My mother and her siblings fought over their family memories once they became drunk. As soon as the adults were drunk the fighting began and, as kids, we were never sure what it was all about, but it always happened. They would start yelling and swearing at each other, and then people would start to leave. Sometimes the table was overturned, or the Christmas tree was pulled down, and once my aunt went upstairs to jump from the balcony.

Alcohol increased the level of damage that could be inflicted on the inhabitants of our house. I became trapped in that house, trying to convince my mother that I was worth being her child and hoping she wouldn't just discard me.

My family was Irish Catholic, and we lived in the poorer areas of Ottawa. We lived mostly in the center town areas, Florence Street, Bell Street, Rochester Street, and Percy Street. I would discover later in life in an article on the settlement of Bytown, Ottawa, that this was where the Catholic people were allowed to settle. The French Catholics and the Italian Catholics also lived in these areas. It included Gladstone, Somerset, Bronson and Mechanicsville/LeBreton Flats. The Centertown area had mostly older, unrenovated houses in need of repair. My mother tried to find places where we could have a yard. We didn't have a lot. Life was rough for her after my father left because he didn't provide anything to help her with the cost of raising three kids on her own.

I had reasons to worry because she had left me a few times. Shortly after my father left, she left me with my paternal grandmother, who had not been a big part of our lives. I was there for some time before she returned for me. I was five at the time.

Another time, she had all three of us pack our bags, and she left us with our little suitcases sitting in a park after saying social services would be by to pick us up. We were there for over an hour before she came back. I was seven at the time.

I do believe that my mother was seriously considering giving us up that day. I believe she went home and thought about it for a while. I believe that's why she had us pack our suitcases and why we were left there for so long. She came back and got us. I never felt safe again. I knew she could get rid of me any time she wanted to.

When I was thirteen, she left me on a farm all summer alone and refused to let me come home even though I begged her to allow me. I became forever terrified that she would eventually get rid of me. I became riddled with shame and self-loathing for having been such a horrible burden to her. The things she said to me deeply damaged my sense of self and damaged my ability to feel OK in the world and among other people. I would never feel acceptable. I would always believe others would reject me because if my own mother hadn't wanted me, then who would?

The places that we were left weren't always the best places, and this can often be the problem when you have a single parent, and they don't have the resources to have you taken care of. The farm we spent so many summers at had its downfalls and we didn't always share these with my mother or anyone else for that matter. I witnessed and experienced incidents of physical abuse that included whippings and beatings. I would never have revealed these for fear of not being believed and then having to return the following year and having to face repercussions for telling. As a child you do not have any power, and so you know enough to keep quiet.

I was once thrown headfirst into a wall while being held by my pants and my shirt. It was the woman who ran the caring of the children who stayed there, and she was not to be crossed. She was a lot harder on her own granddaughter and grandson.

When there are a lot of people drinking in a house, there is a lot of danger of adults behaving inappropriately with children as well. In my family it was the women who tended to behave more inappropriately. We had two Aunts that you literally had to run from, and I recall a number of us holding a door shut with an aunt on the other side trying to push it open to get at us. If she did get a hold of you, she would engage in very inappropriate kissing and grabbing.

Children are the most damaged individuals when alcohol or drugs become part of the family's coping system. Children do not have the capacity to make sense of what is happening or to protect their fragile egos from the raging of an addicted person. They will try to make sense, but the story they create to make sense will often be a very damaging one.

In my family, I believed that I had somehow destroyed my family by being born. It was the only way I could make sense of why my mother didn't want me. I had to have done something wrong. I carried a huge sense of guilt and shame around this sense of responsibility for my family's difficult situation. I felt my father left because of me. I was somehow the straw that broke the camel's back.

My mother's rage at me began just after my father left when I was about five years old. It was also the time that she began to tell me and my relatives that she would die when I turned nineteen. I thought I became for my mother some symbol of the destruction of her dreams of a happy married life. It seemed that at five years of age, I had single-handedly managed to become the cause of my family's disintegration. It was a burden that I would carry for a large part of my life and not one I could talk about because of the shame that came with it.

I wanted to describe this because it is the children who never get a voice in all of this. When my parents became involved in physical disputes, my mother would have my brother take us down the street to the neighbor's place until it was over. She knew how to hide the family dysfunction from social services. When the police arrived, there would be no children present. She protected her own interests but not those of her children because we had already witnessed part of the fight.

The fear that sat with each of us as we sat at the neighbor's house was already happening while we sat there waiting. When one parent says they are going to kill the other, a child has no way of knowing whether this will in fact happen. How were we to be sure that one, or both, wouldn't end up dead? We would have to wait until the call came for us to come back home to know if my mother was still alive.

I'd like you to consider this when we look at children who have a hard time paying attention in school. If you don't know if one of your parents will kill the other, how easy do you think it would be to learn math or any subject for that matter? How do you concentrate when you are sitting with that kind of worry, and you don't know what awaits you when you get home? How hard would it be to sit still and be quiet? I did well in school because I had nothing else to do. Having no friends meant I had a lot of time alone. I ended up doing homework just to have something to do. Nonetheless, it's well worth asking when we see disruptive kids in the classroom.

My sister and brother were not much older than me. When my father left, I was five, my sister was six, and my brother was eight. Although my father left at about this time, he had been coming and going for many years. He had never been a reliable or responsible parent. He stole any money he could get his hands on, even if it meant his children went hungry. My mother would tell many stories of my father's antics when drinking after he had gone.

This would be the only presence I ever had of my father in my life other than the day I walked in on him in bed with the babysitter. I was three at the time, and he kicked the door in my face so hard the doorknob knocked me out. I would be told a story about how I had gotten a concussion when I was three when some kid threw a stone and hit me in the head.

I remember the last time I ever saw him, as if somehow it had become burned in my mind by the fact that he never returned. I watched him walk down Florence Street towards Percy Street. There would be many times I stared back up that street wondering if he would ever come walking back down it. I didn't know enough about the unfolding events to know what was happening. It would only be later, through my mother's stories, that I would piece together where my father went that day and why.

My mother never told us that my father had left for good. That was up to us to somehow figure it out and the level of anger she had when she spoke about him told us not to ask any questions. Eventually you just realized that he wasn't coming back this time. Pieces of the story would tumble out when she was drinking though, and eventually I would fit them together like a puzzle to figure out what happened.

He'd committed a jewelry robbery, and he had been on trial for it. She told us how the police came and that they tore our place apart looking for the jewelry, just when my mother was making supper. She had been peeling potatoes from a fifty-pound bag when they arrived. They made a mess because they just turned drawers upside down in their search. After they left, my mother said she went back to peeling the potatoes, and when she reached in, she found the jewelry in the bag and called the police back to collect it.

She had had enough of him by that point. She wanted him out of her life because all he did was make things more difficult by stealing money from her. She would try hiding the money, but she said he could smell it out. He would run before the end of the trial, and he would not return. All he would leave behind was the bitterness in my mother's heart and the awful aftermath his leaving left his children in.

He would never play a meaningful part in our lives again. He would never contribute a penny to help raise us. He would leave my sister with a terrible aching hole because he had allowed her to believe that she was his princess. He had doted on her just enough to make his leaving a pain that she could never heal from. For years all of the pictures that she appeared in showed a crying child.

His leaving would set the stage for a lifetime of discord between my sister and my mother because my sister came to believe that my mother had driven him away. They would fight right up to my mother's death, adding one more reason for a yelling match in a house that already had far too many reasons. It would leave my sister deeply scarred when her mother died, and an aunt would tell her she drove her mother to her grave.

Despair drove my mother to her grave. She died of addiction and a broken heart. Addiction ensured there would be no chance to recover, and the hurt would just ferment into something stronger over the years. There can be no healing in an addicted family. There can only be bitterness and resentment that emerges every time intoxication loosens the tongue. The remaining actors in this play are left playing out the tragedy forever. In addicted homes, the family members become combatants for the little that's left over after the dysfunction has burned away anything that was good.

Each child will carry their own take on what has occurred in the family. When insanity is part of the world they have grown up with, then the interpretations can be very different.

We each hold selective memories that stand out for us. We each spend different moments with each other that we don't all share. Each of the relationships are different, and loyalties vary depending on these relationships and the events that take place over time. Events can set up resentments, dysfunction can set up unhealthy relationships, and roles can be turned on their heads.

In my family, my sister and mother had an impaired relationship because of my father's leaving. My sister interpreted the event of my father leaving and my mother's bitterness as evidence that my mother forced him to leave and, therefore, she must have hated my sister. She would often claim that my mother didn't love her. My mother would try to prove that she did by giving in to my sister's demands and wants, but of course material goods can't repair the pain.

My sister rebelled against my mother at every turn. This created a crazy pattern that played out over and over while my brother and I tried to manage it without absolutely hating my sister. When you don't know what is going on behind people's behaviors, it just seems like one more aspect of insanity. This can feel like unfairness and set siblings up against each other while really, it's all about the family pain playing itself out over and over. I realized a lot of this years later while I went through my own therapy and education around addiction and its effects on the family. While it was happening, I just could not understand what the hell was going on.

Nothing I can say can adequately explain what it was like to live in the middle of this wounded family. The pain was tangible on most days. I walked around like the house was covered with landmines, fearful of setting off another explosion. The level of yelling was unbearable, and I could find no escape. My mother wanted an audience, and I couldn't get away. My brother and sister learned to stay out of the house as much as possible, but they would have to come home eventually.

Other relatives came and went out of this mess, and the fights went on forever. I once stood outside in forty-below weather because I couldn't take the yelling. It was a day when the hairs inside your nose would freeze with each breath. A friend of my sister took pity on me and took me to her house because she reckoned I would freeze to death if I just stood outside all night. For years afterwards, I was deeply affected anytime I was around people yelling. For a long time, I felt like I was yelling even when I wasn't. I also picked up the habit of yelling and fighting every time I was drunk.

I had no friends. My mother's complete and total destruction of my self-esteem made making friends impossible for me. I couldn't imagine for a minute that anyone could ever like me. How could someone like a person whose own mother didn't want them? As time went by, she used the desire I had to find a way to get her to love me by doing things for her, into a full-time job. She eventually isolated me from any chance I could have to have a friend. I became her full-time companion, her bodyguard, the person who carried whatever she bought, who ran any errands she wanted me to run and, eventually, I became her drinking partner. I was privy to all of her sadness, her suicidal thoughts and her anger.

At some point I became my older brother and sister's parent, and she often held me responsible for my sister's defiant behavior. At thirteen she held me responsible for my sister's pregnancy because I had not told her. I had no way of knowing because I had no knowledge of pregnancy at that point in my life. She kept yelling at me that I knew and that I hadn't told her, and now it was too late for her to have an abortion. She went on for some time about this as if I could have done anything.

She also left me to guard the house after there had been a break-in while she and my two siblings went to an aunt's funeral. I was thirteen and her youngest child, so why was I the one selected to guard the house? I sat there in a chair near the basement door with a butcher knife and a crowbar, absolutely terrified of what I would do if the robbers came back. This is the other aspect of addicted families. They make absolutely no sense. How did my mother come to view her youngest child as her parental partner?

On one occasion she took me to my aunt's place because her boyfriend was beating her up. She went there to confront the boyfriend. How did she think taking me into that situation was in any way helpful? I would have been about twelve years old at the time.

On another occasion, one of my sister's boyfriends, who was a well-known violent criminal, assaulted my sister and mother by throwing a beer bottle through the glass window in our front door while they were standing behind it. My sister received stitches to a cut very near her eye as a result. My mother decided to take me to his house the next day to confront him. I would have been fifteen at the time. Again, what the hell was she thinking? I have to assume that she never gave it much thought. She could not see me as the child I was, but only as what she wanted me to be for her.

There were times when she sent me for things or had me carry things she had bought that, as a girl, were near impossible for me to carry. On one occasion I was expected to carry boxes of floor tiles seven or more blocks to our house. Another time, I tried to manage three paper grocery bags full of groceries the distance of about twelve or more blocks home. I had to hold the two outer bags tightly pressed together to manage the third that was held between them. When one bag ripped, I was beside myself as to what I was supposed to do.

I sometimes felt completely overwhelmed by trying to accomplish things I was not physically strong enough to manage. With my mother there was never an opportunity to say I can't, or I don't want to. If she asked you to do something, you had to just do it.

I remember she sent me up to the bathroom one evening when she was having a family gathering. My aunt had passed out in the bathroom, and no one could use it as a result. My aunt was very heavy, and I was somehow supposed to pull her out from under the tub and drag her to her bedroom.

Finally, another aunt came up to give me a hand because there was no way I would have been able to manage this alone. I ask myself again why she could not see me as the child that I was rather than some other figure she had made me out to be.

She was also unable to realize that I was, in fact, a girl because she just ignored what that meant. She provided nothing to prepare me or help me with the transformation into puberty, including providing any of the essential needs that come with that. She left me in an untenable situation that only further isolated me from my peers and left me in a state of miserable shame. With no bra, underwear or supplies for my period, I found myself in a nightmare of ridicule and shame. At thirteen, I wanted to die because I couldn't bear the pain of living in the world.

This is the gift of addiction: you need to understand that there are twenty-four hours in a day, and 365 days in a year, to really understand how long the sentence is for children caught in the prison of addicted families. I get it that the ideal situation is to have families stay together, but when that becomes a life sentence for children neglected and left with their needs ignored, it can be a very painful beginning to life.

The other thing my mother did was wake me at 1:00 or 2:00 in the morning when my sister hadn't come home, and I was made to get up, get dressed and walk the streets until I either found my sister or her rage subsided. Often my sister would be at one of the places we visited, but they would deny she was there, and then after we left, she would go home and go to sleep.

When my mother and I got home, she would not wake her up, having satisfied the venting of all her anger with me. She would also try and put me into a fight by asking me to take sides with her or my sister. This was a no-win situation because I was damned no matter what I did. Addicted families often set the members of the family up against each other.

Every man for himself was the creed. There was little space for loyalty.

I was a deep kid. Loneliness probably caused this. So many hours alone had left me plenty of time to read and think. The world made absolutely no sense, but I spent plenty of time trying to make sense of it anyway.

I wrote for a time about how I was feeling because I had no one to talk to. My mother found one of these entries and concluded I was off in the head. I accidentally overheard her talking to my brother and sister in the basement about the fact that I might be crazy, and they might have to send me to see a psychiatrist. They agreed with her. I felt extremely threatened by this.

I thought she was planning to have me taken away and locked up somewhere. It was the last time I ever wrote down what was going on with me. It was also the first time I realized that I was totally alone in the world. No one had my back. I was expendable at any point. I was eleven at the time.

Again, I am hoping I am conveying to you the level of constant threat that I lived under. At eleven years of age, I thought I was a loser and that I would die a loser. No child should ever believe this to be true. This is what addicted families do. They destroy the lives of their children. My mother never beat me, although she threatened me enough times for me to think it was a possibility. She would draw her arm back while standing over me and tell me she was going to bash me in the face. She sounded pretty convincing to me.

What she did was psychologically destructive. Bit by bit she destroyed any chance I had to feel like I belonged in the world. When she realized that she had managed to train me to be her devoted servant, she used this to her advantage. If I found a friend, she would end that quickly by accusing me of not giving a damn about her and of being just like my brother and sister.

My mother knew how to hurt you with words. When she was angry her rage was devastating. She could make your life painful, and she had the ability to rage for hours on end. She used guilt to control me. Eventually I could only sense her and her feelings and not my own. I had become completely enmeshed with my mother.

It's also important to note that I loved my mother deeply. She had been my only parent, and I had been so fearful as a child that I clung to the belief that I could get her to love me back. I saw her as the victim of terrible circumstances that left her a single parent stuck in poverty, and that robbed her of having a happy life.

We children were the weight that hung around her neck and, somehow, it was my job to alleviate this weight. I had been the one too many that had made the situation untenable. Somehow, I had to make up for this.

Once, I found my mother face down on the floor in the dining room, and I tried to wake her, but I got no response. I was eleven at the time and there was no one else at home. I didn't know what to do. There was no 911 at that time, and you would not just go and get a neighbor, so I tried calling my uncle, but the phone was busy. It was January and it had been snowing quite a bit, but I decided the best thing would be to go and get him. He lived about seven or eight blocks away.

I set out at a run, running down the middle of the road where there was less snow, down Maclaren, across Bronson, and then down Christie Street. While I was running, I saw this little old lady wipe out on the sidewalk. I ran over, helped her up, wiped the snow off her, asked her if she was OK and then ran off again.

I made it to my uncle's place on Bell Street and got him to come back with me. He managed to wake my mother and got her up into a chair. She didn't seem very happy to see him, and he left shortly afterwards. She then laid into me. She was really pissed that I had gone to get my uncle. She yelled at me for quite some time about doing that, but what she never seemed to really get was that I thought she was dead. I thought my mother was dead and I didn't know what to do. I didn't know what to do if you found your mother dead. No one had ever explained that to me.

Once, when I was thirteen, I was coming home and, as I came down Somerset Street, I was about two blocks from my street when I could hear a commotion ahead. I started hoping it wasn't my family but, as I got closer, I could see that it was.

My mother was trying to run in front of moving cars, trying to get herself hit while my sister was standing on the corner screaming and crying. As I got there, I tried to get my mother to stop doing that and come home, but she wouldn't listen to me and kept saying she was going to kill herself. I had no idea how this got started, and I didn't know how to stop it.

I ran home to see if my brother was home, and he was, so I asked him to help me because Mom was trying to kill herself and could he come and try and get her to stop. He came up to the corner and asked her if she had made his lunch for the next day. I just looked at him because I thought he was crazy, but she said no. He asked her if she would mind coming home and making it before she killed herself and, damn it, she did. She came home and she didn't go back. Nobody talked about it, and I never could figure it out, but I was glad it was over. No one ever talked about anything, ever.

The single most destructive event of my entire life was the fact that my mother predicted her death on my nineteenth birthday when I was five years old and then died a month and a day before I turned nineteen. I will never forget my aunt Dot responding to my mother saying, "Oh my God, Milli, you can't say that to a child."

My mother believed that it was her duty to raise us and that once we were adults, we would just abandon her, and she would end up alone. It was the reason she chose my nineteenth birthday as the date of her death. She would call me into the dining room in front of all my relatives and say, "When she's nineteen, I'm going to die," and she did this every year from the time I was five years old. I was the youngest, and I would be an adult by then and, of course, I would also abandon her.

She made me aware of this belief and I then spent my young life trying to prove that I would not abandon her. It was the perfect trap. I could get her to love me if I gave up my childhood for her. It was an awful price to pay.

I entered her world and carried her despair and anger inside me. I lost my childhood, and despite this awful sacrifice, she still died a month and a day before I turned nineteen. I felt like I had been the clock ticking down to her death. Each year that brought me closer to nineteen made that reality ever more difficult. At her funeral, many aunts reminded me of her prediction and marveled at how close she had come to my actual birthday. I did not need to be reminded of this because I had lived with it since I was five years old.

Parents say things and then never realize what their words do to their children. As children we are not able to decipher what a parent means when they say something like my mother said to me. We attempt to understand, but our limits leave us with an interpretation that can be more damaging than the real meaning of what was said. Today I understand what motivated my mother to say what she said, but as a child, my interpretation was the painful realization that I had somehow destroyed her life.

Parents also believe that their children will forget what happened when they were children or what was said to them. Believe me when I tell you that they do not forget. I remember exactly what my mother said to me. She said, "I needed you as much as I needed two heads; why I ever had you, I'll never know." Those words would echo in my mind throughout my childhood and become a shadow over my adult life as well.

Growing up with the kind of awful binds that addicted parents put their children in is extremely damaging. Children are being raised in these very unhealthy environments that teach them a variety of rules that work against them. Addicted homes teach their children to keep silent and never reveal what is actually going on in the home. The rule is without exception. You cannot speak about what is going on in the home. That would be akin to treason. Children are also taught to suppress their feelings. Addicted parents do not want to have to deal with their children's issues. You must ignore your feelings for the sake of your parents' needs and wishes. You also learn that there is no one you can trust, not even your own family members.

In my family you could also not get ill because that was an inconvenience my mother could not afford. She couldn't take time off work, so she could not have an ill child to care for. In the summer we were sent to a farm to avoid having to have a babysitter for us. Sometimes, necessity dictates the decisions a parent makes. My mother struggled with poverty, and so anything that threatened the meager wages she received could not be wasted in emergencies. If one of us was ill, she would have to have a babysitter or take a day off work, and she couldn't do this. She would become incredibly angry at us if we were ill.

We learned to hide if we were ill. I remember my brother making me and my sister promise that we would not tell my mother that he had split open the palm of his hand after sliding down a rope that had a nail in it. Again, from a child's vantage point, the why wouldn't have been understood, and the rule would be one more that seemed confusing. The underlying message would clearly be that you could expect no comfort if you were ill or had hurt yourself. During the stage of childhood illnesses, my mother would put us all together if one of us got an illness like measles. It was easier to handle if we all had measles than if we became ill at different times. Once, when I was seven, I ruptured myself learning to ride a bike, and I didn't want to tell my mother. I hid my pants in the closet, but my sister told her. I was terrified of her finding out.

I also often fell as a kid, and this infuriated my mother because I often tore the knees out of my pants. She couldn't afford clothes for us, so this became another hardship for her. She would yell at me, "What's wrong with you? Don't you know how to walk?"

The difficulties faced by families that have to struggle to manage financially were worsened by my mother's alcoholism and her rage. It was exacerbated by the difficulties of her life. When she couldn't handle things, she would rage at us. We were part of the struggle she faced because she had to feed and clothe us, and pay for all of the bills on top of that. Some people point to the alcohol and say, but she could afford that. That is true, but she used the alcohol as some relief, and even though it never really provided that relief, she returned to it over and over again because that was all she could find.

I would see myself resort to the same flawed reasoning over and over, not knowing what else to do, even though this actually caused me more problems in the long run. It is the insanity of addiction. It initially seems like the answer, and by the time it clearly becomes the problem, you are too addicted and too mentally affected to either make the connection or stop.

After my father left, my mother sat us down and told us that we were to tell people at school, and anyone else who asked, that our father was dead. This was a serious bind for me because we attended Catholic school and lying was a sin. The alternative would be worse, dealing with my mother's wrath. My mother didn't want people to know that my father was a criminal or that he had taken off. This would have brought her unnecessary shame. The trial had already caused her embarrassment because some of the neighbors had to testify in court.

After her death I found a small piece of paper cut out of the newspaper in her wallet that said Robert Byron James no longer resides at 267 Florence Street. I believe, back then, that you had to have this put in the paper for some legal reasons, but the fact that she carried it around with her all those years spoke volumes about how hurt she had been.

I have chosen to write this book because I wanted to shine a light on just how damaging addiction is and to hopefully speak for some of the people who never get considered in our response to this problem. I saw firsthand how addiction could deliver a death blow to any chance of some family peace and joy. I experienced how an addicted parent can destroy the childhood of her children even though that might have been the last thing that she wanted.

I do not believe that my mother set out to deliberately destroy my childhood, but in her addiction, she did so. Addiction creates a very self-centered response to the world. It creates a trap that does not allow people to heal from whatever pain their life has dealt them. Unresolved pain drives addiction, and the pain leaks out in the most destructive ways. I would come to know that personally as well, as my own addiction developed and took over my life and leaked out over the people around me.

I tried alcohol for the first time when I was seven years old. I did not know what it was when I was offered a glass of wine while we were visiting an Italian family that had once lived in the same house as us. They had moved away, and they had invited us to come over for dinner one evening. They offered me a glass of wine, which was, for them, a cultural norm, and I took it and drank it. I believe I had a second glass that evening before my mother headed home with all of us on foot. I was so drunk I couldn't walk right. My mother was very upset because this would not look good if anyone saw us or stopped us. It would be hard to explain why her youngest child was so drunk she could barely walk. I was violently ill when I got home.

The next time I drank, I was thirteen years old. It was relatively easy to drink in my house. My brother had parties in the basement, and he had alcohol, and he gave us some, if we didn't tell my mother he'd brought it into the house. Eventually the lines blurred, and my mother allowed us to drink in the house as long as we didn't go out. I had a problem right off the bat. I couldn't seem to control my drinking. I would drink until long past the point where I should have stopped. The only thing that offered me some control was that I didn't have access every day.

When I was fifteen years of age, my mother wanted a drinking partner. She used to drink with an aunt who had lived with us, but after she moved out, my mother wanted someone to drink with at home. Since I had somehow become her co-parent, she decided it would be me. At first, I didn't really want to drink with her all the time, but she was always very insistent. She would say, "Come on, have a drink with your mother," over and over until I just gave in. It's not like I didn't want to drink alcohol, but I think early on I was aware of how damaging it had been in my family. My mother and my aunt fought continuously, and it was just another source of difficulty I had to put up with as they warred with each other every time they got drunk. These were some of the worst fights that I witnessed, and they both drank far too much when they drank together. This was also the source of information for most of the family's dysfunctional secrets. They spilled out venom as one family member yelled at another.

These kinds of experiences are normal in addicted families, but they are not normal. They are crazy making. These very disturbing incidents played out over and over throughout my life. I was never able to understand this.

Once, my aunt and mother were fighting during Christmas dinner when all my relatives were present, and my aunt stated she was going to jump off the balcony. She headed upstairs and my mother and sister ran outside. My mother yelled up to the balcony that she should hurry up and jump because it was cold outside, and she added that she wasn't going to clean up the mess. This was so distressing for me, but it seemed like I should have considered it just a part of normal behavior. I was looked at as if I was the person that had the problem.

How do children understand the world they are living in when the events taking place in their home make no sense? You can't ask the people involved to help you understand it because they are the people causing it. How do children manage this when they are sworn to secrecy so they can't even ask someone else about what is going on? There is no way to make sense of incidents such as these. These are not normal behaviors, but if you do not have anything to compare them to, then what is normal really?

Understanding Addiction through the Lens of Trauma and the Neuroscience of the Brain

There has been an important study called the Adverse Childhood Experiences Study (ACE Vincent J Felitti 2003). This study shone a light on what fueled the development of addiction in so many people. It concluded that based on the answers to ten items identifying childhood adverse experiences, the higher the score, the more likely people would experience chronic illnesses that would impair and shorten the life span. Addiction was one of those chronic illnesses. As the score went higher, so did the likelihood of addiction. The relationship was so strong that the results were more powerful than any other example of relational studies ever seen. The study was conducted in the 1990s, yet this information has taken its time to be fully understood and accepted as some of the most significant findings in health care to date. It also predicted things like diabetes, heart trouble, obesity, irritable bowel, chronic fatigue, and cancer, among other immune-related illnesses. It makes sense when we realize that people often try to find ways to soothe their stress, and often these include things that are not health promoting, like smoking, using drugs and alcohol, eating unhealthy foods, and lowering physical activity, among others. In Canada, the Alberta Family Wellness Initiative has taken this information to a more active level by launching The Brain Story, a nineteen-module, online, free course that covers all of the most relevant research sparked by this study. One of the focuses of that work is to highlight the need to teach people how to influence the child's brain to develop and grow and to help incorporate resilience into that development. I urge anyone to access this free learning, which is one of the best resources I have seen on combating the negative effects of stress on children. As a health promotion tool, it outdoes itself in the prevention of long-term chronic illnesses in adulthood. When I took the questionnaire, I had a ten out of ten on the list of adverse events. I would say that having addiction in the family puts a person at great risk of scoring high on this questionnaire.

The ACE Studies Vincent J. Felitti 2003
The items that are on the ACE questionnaire include:

Adverse Events:
1. Recurrent physical abuse
2. Recurrent emotional abuse
3. Contact sexual abuse
4. Alcohol and/or drug abuse in household
5. Incarcerated household member
6. Family member chronically depressed, mentally ill or suicidal
7. Mother treated violently
8. One or no parents
9. Physical neglect
10. Emotional neglect.

Resulting Health Risks
1. Cardiovascular disease
2. Cancer
3. Heart Attacks
4. High Blood Pressure
5. Stroke
6. Diabetes

7. Weight Gain
8. Exhaustion
9. Reduced Growth Hormone Levels
10. Compromised Immune Function
11. Bone Loss
12. Addiction
13. Mental illness.

The result of these findings and a more comprehensive biological and neurological understanding of addiction has put us in a unique position to speak about the underlying causes of addiction. It shows once and for all that addiction is not about willpower but about a number of factors coming together that change the nature of the brain's structure and functioning. The Surgeon General's Report on Alcohol, Drugs and Health, published by the U.S. Department of Health and Human Services 2016, called Finding Addiction in America, details this new presentation on how the brain is impacted by addiction and how it changes over time.

What does neuroscience tell us?

There are three areas implicated in addiction.
The Basal Ganglia: involved in Binge/Intoxication
The Extended Amygdala: involved in Withdrawal/ Negative Affect
The Prefrontal Cortex: involved in Preoccupation/ Anticipation.

The Basal Ganglia
Binge/Intoxication

1) Initial use may begin with a moment of impulsivity, the person tries the substance.

2) Continued use depends on the effect of the substance on the person
a) The experience is pleasurable, and so the use is positively reinforced
b) Experience removes something displeasurable, and so the use is negatively reinforced

My personal experience:
When I first tried alcohol, I felt a sense of relief, it was like a deep sigh. It was the first time I didn't feel the overwhelming sense of anxiety of living in my home. It made me feel good and removed the anxiety I was experiencing.

Positive Reinforcement

Could come directly from the effects of the drug:

- The drug experience is enjoyable.

Could come from other consequences of drug use, such as:

- Acceptance from a peer group.
- Being with others.

My personal experience:
I enjoyed the pleasurable effects of drinking and taking drugs. Using drugs or alcohol suddenly gave me access to a peer group. The only thing necessary to belong to this group was the willingness to use drugs or alcohol. I gained instant acceptance through my willingness to use drugs.

Negative Reinforcement

Could come directly from the effects of the drug.

- Relief from painful emotional experiences such as Stress, Anxiety, or Depression.

Could come from other consequences of drug use, such as:

- Relief from social isolation.
- Relief from feelings of being different.

My personal experience:
The alcohol and drugs allowed me to alter my feelings very quickly. It provided relief from the stress of living in my home. I could escape the emotional pain for a period of time. Using also made me feel like I belonged somewhere. I could be with other people, and I wasn't so socially phobic or isolated.

Addiction Hijacks the Brain's Reward System

- The Brain's reward system rewards eating and sex, which ensures the survival of the species through the release of Dopamine, which provides us with a sense of pleasure.
- All drugs of abuse affect this system by prompting the release of Dopamine.
- The brain then equates these drugs with survival.

The Reward System

- Drugs and alcohol activate this system.
- Stimuli associated with drug or alcohol use also activate this system.
- These stimuli become triggers or cues to use and promote substance seeking and substance use.

- The triggers themselves cause a release of Dopamine, which increases the desire to seek the drug.

My personal experience:
When I was in recovery, I became aware of how true this was because if I were exposed to anything that reminded me of using or was associated with using, I would become very irritable or find myself having cravings to use. I once went to have coffee with friends in a restaurant where there was a bar near where we were sitting and, as time went on, I became more and more irritable until I finally realized it was the bar. I often drank in restaurant bars. I had to get up and leave because it was so uncomfortable for me.

Habit Formation and Compulsivity

- The release of Dopamine is reduced in people taking drugs or alcohol.
- The desire for the release of Dopamine causes habit formation because the habit of using is reinforced by the release of Dopamine.
- This habit eventually leads to a compulsion to avoid the negative consequences of not using substances, which is the reduced release of Dopamine.

My personal experience:
The more I used, the more I wanted to use. Eventually, using became more normal than not using. I couldn't function well without it. I never learned how to develop healthy coping strategies. The drug and alcohol use seemed like the solution to my problems. After a while it became the most prominent thing in my mind.

The Extended Amygdala
Withdrawal/Negative Affect

The Brain's Stress System
When activated, it produces:

- Corticotrophin Releasing Factor (CRF)
- Norepinephrine
- Dynorphin

These produce:

- Depression
- Anxiety
- Irritability

Tolerance and Withdrawal

- Tolerance: Drug and alcohol use effects on Dopamine diminish over time, and more is required to achieve the same effect.
- When drugs or alcohol are not taken, there is little release of Dopamine, and the person experiences Anxiety, Depression and Irritability because the stress system is activated.

My personal experience:
My use increased over time in both volume and frequency. It would take more to get the same relief, and I needed to use substances more often because they seemed to wear off sooner. I began to experience withdrawal symptoms like extreme anxiety, depression, and irritability. I couldn't manage how I

was feeling. I would be constantly on edge if I hadn't used. I wanted to crawl out of my own skin. I would fly into rages. I couldn't tolerate the smallest stressors. I was impossible to be around. I had trouble concentrating, my hands would shake, and my head hurt. I had to find something to help me. I often took numerous codeine pills to try and alleviate these symptoms, but the best solution was always to use substances. The key became never to run out of drugs or booze. Despite this, I didn't realize I was addicted. It wouldn't be until I actually tried to stop using that I would realize I was addicted.

The Trap

- Negative feelings that accompany withdrawal strongly motivate continued substance use.
- Taking substances relieves the negative feelings of withdrawal.
- Withdrawal symptoms increase over time.

My personal experience:
There was a point where not using became very painful because I could not stand being without some substance to help me deal with the increasing irritability and depression. Even though my using substances often led to other problems created by being intoxicated, not using had become too painful to manage. This is what I see as the trap because I knew my using was causing problems, but not using seemed to be causing more problems.

The Prefrontal Cortex
Preoccupation/Anticipation

Controls our Executive Functioning:

- The ability to organize thoughts and activities.
- Prioritize tasks, manage time, make decisions.
- Regulate one's actions, emotions, and impulses.

My personal experience:
Eventually, I became preoccupied with using or finding more to use. It's like it suddenly occupied an awful lot of my thinking. I was always thinking of my next opportunity to use and where I was going to get my next score, how much I had left and how much money I had in order to pay for more. It was endless. If my source ran out and I had to wait, it was agonizing. There were times I couldn't get out of bed because I just could not function without anything. I once put a barbell through a wall because I was so irritable.

The Go System/The Stop System

The Go System:

- It is often used to engage in behaviors that help us achieve goals.
- Activity here increases the urge to repeat the behaviors that are pleasurable.
- Increases dramatically in the presence of substance-related triggers or cues.
- Increases the habit response system so that behaviors become automatic and subconscious.

The Stop System:

- Inhibits the activity of the Go System.
- Controls habit responses.

- Reduces the ability of triggers or cues to produce relapses.
- Controls the brain's stress and emotional system.

The Problem:

- People with substance abuse disorders have impairments in executive functioning.
- They have increased activity in the Go System.
- They have decreased activity in the Stop System.
- People with substance abuse disorders and people with PTSD have smaller volume in the Prefrontal Cortex.

Factors that contribute to and affect the development of addiction:

- Genetics
- Mental Health
- Trauma History (ACE Studies)
- Personality
- Social Support
- Sense of Self
- Connection to Others
- Resiliency
- Age of use, length of use, poly-drug use
- Attachment history
- Previous head injury or a compromised brain

My personal experience:
I had a lot of factors that increased my risk for addiction. Both of my parents were addicted, and I had grown up in an addicted family. I had a significant trauma history and scored ten out of ten on the ACE questionnaire. My mental health was compromised by the family I grew up in and by a family history of bipolar disorder. I had an insecure personality from having been told I was unwanted by my mother and having been rejected and bullied by my peers. I had little in the way of social support, and the friends I did cultivate were people who were alcohol and drug abusers. I had an impaired sense of self from feeling unwanted. I had little meaningful connections to anyone. I had little resiliency and saw no other way to tolerate my life other than by using substances. I started active use at the age of thirteen and would use any drug I could get my hands on. I had an impaired and extremely dysfunctional attachment to my mother. I suffered two major concussions, one when I was three and the other when I was thirty. I think, given what I experienced in my life, it would have been odd if I hadn't developed an addiction.

Other Issues

- Adolescents have greater risks associated with use because they have an undeveloped prefrontal cortex.
- Heavy use can affect the development of their brains.
- Those who have more severe long-term use may have had pre-existing differences in the volume of their prefrontal cortex.
- Co-occurring mental health issues are common in people with Substance abuse disorders, particularly PTSD.

Effects of Acute Stress

- Increased Blood Glucose > Excessive insulin secretion, Type II Diabetes.
- Increased Blood Pressure > Hypertension, coronary heart disease.
- Modulation of immune system > Vulnerability to inflammatory diseases, Asthma, Arthritis.
- Reduced Motivation for rewarding stimuli > loss of interest, depression.
- Vigilance and arousal > Hyperarousal and anxiety disorders.
- Consolidation of aversive memories > Preponderance of aversive memories, PTSD.

My personal experience:
The home that I grew up in and the home I lived in during my early adulthood were both extremely stressful. I was a witness to a lot of very disturbing situations because everyone around me was actively using alcohol or drugs or both. When I began using, this added more access to dangerous people and situations. I was constantly in a state of stress because something crazy was always taking place. Using substances at my workplace added to that stress because the place was so dysfunctional, and people's behaviors were so extreme.

The Story of My Own Addiction

I lived with acute stress for the majority of my life prior to recovery. I bounced from one dangerous or distressing experience to another. My own use set me up to be in a world where dangerous things happened. My childhood was impacted by the behavior of the people around me. When I entered recovery, I had a hard time not living in a chaotic world because I was so used to that world that the quiet was difficult for me. It's like you were always waiting for the other shoe to drop. That created another type of anxiety. It was hard to let go of the hypervigilance that developed after living so long in an insane world.

I had a problem with alcohol in that every time I drank, I behaved in ways that left me embarrassed and ashamed. I was filled with undealt pain and hurt. It would come spilling out when I was drunk. I wavered from rage to drunken sobbing. I drank until I blacked out and didn't know what I had done the night before. The anxiety that accompanied the terrible feelings that I had done something I shouldn't have, sent me back to drinking the next morning to drown it out. I acted dangerously and almost killed myself on a number of occasions, once almost careening off the fourteenth-floor balcony of my sister's boyfriend's place after he had served me numerous spiked drinks. I was sixteen at the time.

The problem with all substances that cause a mood alteration is; if you have had a traumatic background, you will go back to it, over and over again, to numb the pain you do not know how to deal with. The trauma of my background made addiction an inevitability. It was a trap, and in my over twenty years of working in the field of addiction counseling, I have seen the same thing over and over. There's no way you see it coming. You try a substance, and you think like everyone else, it's just something to try every now and then, but the trauma sets the hook that snares you, and you just can't escape.

I was caught the first day I took a drink. It would be the nature of my relationship with all drugs of abuse. Each time I looked for a solution, and every time the solution became the problem.

Addiction is a cruel trap because it is born from the pain and hurt the person can't manage to deal with. Sometimes that hurt goes way back to early childhood, and sometimes the traumas come later or just reoccur throughout one's life. The potential for traumatization begins at birth, and some would say that even in the womb we can be damaged by the experiences of the mother, by what she is exposed to, and her level of stress. Certainly, the mother's drug use or alcohol use can have a direct effect on the fetus and the development of the child.

My mother drank regularly, and we were born at a time when concern over a mother's drinking or drug use while pregnant was not as well-known as it is today. I believe that my mother drank during her pregnancy because there would have been no reason not to. This would have added to the likelihood that one or more of her children would be vulnerable to addiction.

Both my brother and I would be addicted to alcohol, and my sister would die from a cigarette smoking addiction. Both my brother and I had a similar response to alcohol. We both resembled my mother when she drank, and we both had a tendency to argue or get into a shouting match.

When your parents are impacted by addiction, you are left exposed to unhealthy ways of interacting, and so that is how you learn to interact as well. The experience leaves you in a position where you are bound to have difficulty in relationships because all you have as an example is this unhealthy model you grew up with. My parents' marriage fell apart, and my father would have two more failed relationships in his life. My brother, my sister, and I all had failed relationships. My brother and sister would go on to each have another relationship.

After a seventeen-year disastrous marriage, I could not do that again. I had never known how to be in a healthy relationship. I had stumbled upon my relationship out of no effort of my own. Left to myself, I would have likely never found my way into a relationship. I had been so damaged by my relationship with my mother, and her negative effect on my self-esteem and sense of female gender, that I would not have known how to attract a guy.

I was set up on a date with my husband, and he was as inadequate at relationships as me. A perfect match for failure and, of course, we failed miserably. I was seventeen when I met my husband, and he introduced me to drugs. This would become more of a problem for me than for him. His problem would be alcohol and an inability to express his emotions. We would never be able to resolve our relationship problems.

Desperation caused me to hang onto the man I met on a blind date. I had no illusions. This might be my only chance to have a relationship, and he came around as my mother was caught in her battle with cancer. I needed another person to hang onto for dear life. My mother was dying, and I would soon be alone in the world. This might be my only chance to secure a connection with somebody else.

It was doomed to fail from the beginning. It was built on what had happened to me with my mother. I would not see that I had chosen the same dysfunction again because, of course, I was blind to it. This is one of the sad realities of having grown up in an abusive home; you are bound to keep choosing the same thing because it feels familiar, and somehow, we equate familiarity with safety. We don't see the trap until we have firmly stepped into it, and then we don't know how to get out. I couldn't see that the man I eventually chose to marry didn't know how to express his feelings, which meant he couldn't tell me that he loved me. He would never even compliment me. I could try as hard as I wanted to, and he would never leave me feeling that I was truly loved.

This applies to other areas of our lives as well. The first full-time job I had was in a provincial bank. I would be part of that work environment for over thirteen years, and it was as dysfunctional as an addicted family. I worked there for a few years while my mother was ill and, for a short time, after she died. I left to go to school to take Fine Arts in college. I also left because the manager who was working there was an alcoholic and he was terrorizing the staff. He eventually would be charged with embezzling the bank's money.

I returned to the bank after college because there was no getting a job in the arts. The old manager was gone but the one that would eventually replace him was a winner. He was another alcoholic. It didn't take long, and it was an alcoholic workplace. When I first started back, people were going out for lunch and drinking and then going out after work and continuing to drink. At first, I couldn't understand how they managed to come to work the next day after drinking all evening. I found out when one of the guys produced a bag full of uppers.

I had already been exposed to a number of different drugs by then. I used pot almost daily, and eventually it would be daily. I'd also used cocaine, mescaline, uppers, heroin, and hallucinogens. My drug use followed the trends in what was available at any time. If it was a drug, then I wanted to use it.

The first time I used chemical drugs, I remember feeling

like I wanted to feel like that forever. It was still about the escape for me. I hated being sober and without some chemical in me. That's the defining aspect of addiction; normal is just not tolerable. Living in me was unbearable. I felt like I wanted to crawl out of my skin. Once I discovered that I could take drugs and suddenly change the way I felt and gain some distance from my internal pain, I never wanted to go back.

If I couldn't find any drugs, then I had to drink, and that was always dangerous because I had absolutely no control over alcohol if that was all I had available to me. Smoking pot allowed me to control my drinking, so I actually knew when to stop drinking. Uppers, on the other hand, made things much more dangerous because then I would continue to drink, and I wouldn't pass out. This often led to violent behavior. There were a couple of times when I assaulted people, and thankfully, they were people that I knew, and they knew it was the alcohol and not me. I always said that alcohol chose me, and I chose drugs. Alcohol would always be my undoing. I could not predict what I would do under its effects.

The bank continued to become more and more dysfunctional as time went by. At least five of us were involved in dysfunctional drinking, including the manager, the accountant, and the assistant manager. The farther things disintegrated, the more damaging the relationships became. Those who didn't drink alcohol became the codependents of those who did.

The codependent staff would cover for the manager, who spent from noon on out drinking in a bar. Head Office, which was in Oshawa, would call, and the secretary would say he was busy with a client, and he'd call them back. She'd then call the bar and tell him Head Office had called. He'd come back and call them and then go back to the bar after he finished the call. The management staff were also fighting with each other, because no one wanted to be the only senior staff member left behind while the others were out drinking all afternoon, because somebody had to remain in the office due to having the combinations to access the vault and the cash.

Depending on who you were allied with, you could also be out drinking with one of them. These disputes pitted people allied with any of the three senior people against each other. The dysfunction just escalated as relationships with these three people broke down. It was as dysfunctional and, in some ways, more dysfunctional than my family of origin. Insanity was still a daily part of my life.

Absolutely inappropriate things would take place in the bank. One time the manager chased people around with the fire extinguisher, spraying it at people. He managed to send the framed interest rate sign flying across the customer area's floor, where the glass in it smashed. At Christmas time he would be drinking in his office, and he'd offer a number of the customers a drink.

On one occasion he began grabbing my breasts, and the rest of the staff took off out the door because it was the end of the day. They left me with this guy grabbing me, and at one point I had lifted a stool up to hold it in front of me and keep him away. He began unscrewing the base of the stool to get at me. He then followed me into the vault, grabbed me from behind, and pulled me to the floor. It totally flipped me out. I managed to get up and I was yelling at him to stay away from me and to keep his hands off of me. The assistant manager was still there and saw me exit the vault and grab my coat to head for the door. Three times the manager tried to stop me from leaving before I managed to get out the door. I think he realized he'd done something wrong and was trying to make a joke of it. I was really scared at the time, and I just wanted to get out of the office.

The following Monday, when he was away on holiday, I asked the staff about what they had seen, and they denied seeing anything. They had been content to leave me with this guy attacking me and then denied they saw anything. If this isn't the perfect example of dysfunction, I don't know what is. The staff were all women, and none of them were close to the manager. They just didn't want to be involved.

I ended up taking the security video because part of the attack would have been recorded. When I left the night of the attack, I had been shaking because I hadn't seen that coming, and it really frightened me. I think what was even more frightening was that nobody I worked with was willing to help me or seemed to care about what had happened to me. The other frightening thing was my own husband didn't seem to care either. I'd left a piece of jewelry on my counter that I wanted to go back and get, and I asked him if he would go with me, and he said no. Even though I was shaking, he didn't care.

My relationship had also been adding some more craziness to my life. After my mother died, my sister invited my boyfriend to move in with us, into the rental home we had been living in, with my mother. Shortly after this, she invited his sister to move in. I hadn't really wanted to stay in that house and was planning to move out, but my sister seemed to have other plans I was unaware of. My sister left not long after, and I was left with the remnants of my mother's belongings, which were, for the most part, items that needed to be thrown away.

I also had to contend with the behavior of my boyfriend's sister, who was caught up in addiction as well. She was in a hurry to burn herself out as fast as possible, and drugs and alcohol were a big part of that. She would bring the police to our door more than a few times, with behaviors that were fueled by her addiction.

She assaulted a friend's mother on one occasion. Once, the homicide detectives came to pick her up because she left a threatening message, cut from words from the newspaper, on the door of her friend's neighbor because they had complained about the late-night noise and partying. It was like being back in my family of origin, complete with the crazy, unpredictable behaviors.

My future husband and I lived on the third floor, which we had made into a small apartment for ourselves. The behavior of his sister was so problematic that we had to run a microphone down through the heating registers from the third floor to the first floor living room in order to monitor the craziness.

She tied the door to our place to the railing one time after leaving a message saying she was going to poison my pet rabbit, again using words cut out of the newspaper. This is more evidence of just how crazy the behavior of addicted people can be. She would often go out drinking and pick up some guys with her friend. They would then claim they were going to the bathroom and leave, after the guys had spent considerable money on them paying for their drinks.

She once woke up with someone in bed with her that she did not know, nor did she remember coming home with. These were things the average person would never think would happen.

The people you associate with when you are using drugs can be every bit as crazy. She brought some dangerous people to our house on more than one occasion. My husband's sister would die at the age of thirty-two from cancer. It was a tragedy that would leave two very young children without a mother and with a father who was so addicted he would struggle to care for them. It wouldn't be the first time I saw addiction set a family up to lose.

Later in my relationship, I began to create associations with dealers because I wanted to use drugs even though my husband did not. That was not always the safest thing, depending on who you managed to get involved with.

At first, I bought from people that I knew were friends, but eventually you end up with different connections. I bought drugs from a biker gang member for a while, and I remember having to go through a window onto a fire escape to get away when he was threatening to collect a drug debt from a friend, whose place I was at.

Drugs always brought you farther into a more dangerous world. My husband and I were once trapped in a kitchen at a party, where two big guys were threatening another friend with a butcher knife. They kept stabbing the knife into a beer case, saying that was what they intended to do with him. The other guy was blocking the door so we couldn't leave.

The guy they had chosen to intimidate was a fellow who had been hit by a truck as a young boy and this had forever affected him. If you met him, it wouldn't take long to realize that there was something not quite right. These guys knew that as well. It was why they chose him to do this to. We were just captive spectators.

It was a very traumatizing experience for me. It tapped into the many times I was bullied as a child at school, because I was poor and often dressed poorly and often smelled. Because no one intervened in my situation, I was left at the mercy of all those who enjoyed bullying others. This situation just tapped into my barely suppressed rage.

I began saying things to them that could have resulted in us having the tables turned on. I was so angry. My husband kept kicking me under the table, trying to get me to shut up. We eventually got out of there with our friend.

I realized I had not managed to take one step away from my history of growing up in an addicted family. I had managed to find an addicted workplace and joined up with an addicted boyfriend and his addicted sister. I was immersed in the addicted world, and I could not get away from it. The first nineteen years were spent with my mother, and the next fifteen would be spent in an addicted workplace and an addicted relationship. When this is all you know, then this seems like the norm. I couldn't see anything else.

I could give you all the details of the events that took place in these places and this would read like a rather dark comedy. The reality though is that it was never funny, and, most often, very stressful and toxic.

At the bank, I came to a point where I did not want to go on. My husband was entirely money-focused, and he did not care about how sick my workplace was. I would come to the end of each day in a barely contained state of rage. The craziness with which people interacted in this work environment made every day a nightmare.

One manager acted out her rage on one employee after another, only moving on to the next when she had reduced one to tears. When she had done this to everyone, she began all over again.

The main manager took pleasure in stirring up a mentally unwell client who was about six feet tall and carried a knife in his sock. He would say something to rile him up and then just walk away and watch the teller try to deal with the aftermath.

Depending on which one of the managers was ruling that day, different people were given breaks, while others were left to do all the work. The animosity between the employees was palpable at times.

This so resembles the addicted family, it's uncanny. I had managed to find a place to work that would just continue the abuse I had experienced as a child. At times, I would become so despondent that I just wished someone would come in to rob the bank, and I was going to say, "Go on; make my day." I teetered on the brink of suicidal and homicidal thoughts. I had spent too many years in the world of addiction, which made no sense whatsoever, and where people acted unpredictably cruel.

My mind was affected by living for such a long time in situations that were made extreme by addiction. I saw too much. I experienced too much. It was one crazy situation after another, and I either played the leading role or I was victimized by someone else's insanity.

I had numerous situations where I was threatened sexually. At thirteen, I was locked in a basement by my sister with a twenty-seven-year-old guy who attacked me sexually. This was repeated with a thirty-two-year-old guy when I was sixteen.

Once, when I was with my boyfriend at his friend's rooming house, I was blocked in a bathroom by a guy who threatened to rape me. Another time, when I was at a friend's place from work, her brother grabbed me inappropriately when we had all gone for a walk.

These kinds of things were not uncommon, which again led to the belief that reality was pretty twisted. The other problem is that no one seemed to be very disturbed by them. How can anyone make sense of this?

My life was splattered with acts of craziness that could not be made sense of. If this was normal, then living had become impossible to tolerate. Suicide entered my life and became a constant companion for a very long period. It eventually occupied every single day and every single night. Sometimes it was accompanied by homicidal thoughts as I came to see myself as trapped in a world with people bent on inflicting as much hurt as possible.

My husband had some strange infatuation with guns, and we had many assault rifles in the house, including an AK47 with a foldable stock. It was not the best thing to have access to, and I entertained some pretty serious thoughts that I thankfully never acted out. There was a point where I began to realize that I needed some help if I was going to survive.

My marriage went consistently downhill. I chose not to

have any children because I knew that I couldn't possibly raise a child without causing the same damage that had been caused to me. My husband would also not have made a very good parent at that time either. He was unable to feel anything. He had one interest in me which was sexual and beyond that, he acted in ways that told me that I didn't matter to him in the least.

In my own anger and recklessness, I hurt him many times psychologically. I would try to make it work until his lack of care for me would drive me to attack him when I was drunk. I would eventually feel guilty and try once again to make it work, but it could not possibly work. We were not healthy enough and addiction ran through our relationship. He was more of a drinker than a drug user in the latter half of our relationship, but the effect was the same. You cannot be in a healthy relationship when addiction is in the picture. We grew further and further apart until we could barely tolerate each other. At some point going to treatment became the chance to get away from both my work and my home life.

The other thing that addiction does is put you at risk for a mental health issue. I developed bipolar disorder. I'm not sure when it first emerged, but I do remember being severely depressed from a very young age. Given the home I was raised in, I'm not surprised that I would have become depressed. You can't go on and on while being continually disparaged without becoming depressed.

I was eleven when I first remembered being really sad all of the time. By the time I had careened out of control with my addiction, I was suicidal on a daily basis. It's all I could think of. I so hated my life at that point, that every day had become a painful existence that I no longer wanted. This was what finally made me seek some help. I either had to get some help or I had to kill myself.

I had tried to stop using substances on my own, but I could not do this. I couldn't make it through a single day without using something. It was the first time I realized that I was addicted. If you never try to stop, you don't know that you can't. You still think you have a choice. If I was going to try and change my life, I needed someone else's help to do it. This forced my hand and brought me into contact with addiction treatment. It would change the rest of my life.

The first time I went to ask for help I was not able to follow through because I was too afraid. I hadn't trusted anyone in my life because there had been no one to trust. My doctor had made an appointment for me with a psychologist because I was extremely suicidal. I thought they would try and brainwash me somehow, and I wasn't up for that.

I had lived so long in the abnormal that I was afraid of actually getting help, because I didn't even know what that looked like, and I was so sure that they would just be another person who would hurt me. My family thought I was crazy, so what if I was?

It was recommended that I see a family counselor, and perhaps my husband and I could do some marriage counseling. I saw an addiction doctor, but when he mentioned residential treatment that was just too scary for me.

My husband refused to go to counseling, so I went by myself. The agreement was that I wasn't to use any drugs during the time I was getting counseling. It was recommended after a few sessions, that I leave my husband and leave my job.

I was terrified of finding myself unable to support myself and ending up in poverty. I had grown up in poverty, and I had been traumatized by that. It was tied up with the death of my mother.

When my mother became ill, I was sixteen years old, and she would die one month and one day before my nineteenth birthday. She had worked all of her life as a lab technician in a dairy. She had never missed a day in twenty-five years. When she tried to get unemployment insurance she was refused because she had a fatal illness. We had little money to live on because women were not paid much money at that time, regardless of the job they did. Our lives had been defined by poverty, and during this time of her illness, things just became worse.

At one point we faced Christmas without any food, and if it weren't for the people she worked with we would have gone without, while my mother lay in a bed with cancer. She eventually got her unemployment payments, but they made her go to the office, where she would have to wait for over an hour to be seen. Despite the pain she was in, she had to do this, in order to get each and every check.

We had always been poor. Someone would drop off clothes donations to us every now and then. We watched a little portable black and white TV. I would be given the job of painting the pattern into the rug that had become threadbare over time. We had little in the way of possessions.

At one point she appealed to welfare when she hadn't been able to get anything from unemployment insurance. They came to the house, and I was told this was to see if we had anything we could sell. Of course, we didn't. They offered to lend my mother two hundred dollars that she would have to pay back. She declined. It was traumatizing to me to see how the system treated my mother.

Two weeks before she would die, she called an ambulance to go to the hospital, and they refused, saying she had a known illness. We had never owned a car, and we had never taken a bus. We walked everywhere. We had certainly never been able to take a taxi. Looking back, I now see that they expected her to find her own way to the hospital. At that moment, the problem seemed insurmountable. It was the first time I saw my mother with a look of terror on her face. She had rarely let the veil of toughness fall, but two and a half years of cancer had broken her.

Over several calls, she pleaded with them until she finally said, "If I die here in front of my children, it will be on your head." They came but they refused to bring in a stretcher, so she had to walk out to the ambulance even though she was weak and had great difficulty walking.

At the hospital they refused to adequately manage her pain. I would ask them to give her something because she was almost delirious with the pain, and they would refuse because it wasn't time yet. She was going to die, and nothing could change that, but still they refused.

It was devastating to me to watch all this unfold while I was losing my only parent. This was the mother that I had tried so hard to prove to her, that I would never abandon her. It left a deep rage inside of me, and it scarred me deeply.

Given what I had experienced, I never believed that there was anyone out there who would ever care about me. Asking for help was a desperate move, and I held little faith in the system that had discarded my mother with such callousness.

I was terrified of leaving the job I hated without having an alternative because I knew my husband did not want to support me, and I feared the system would treat me the same way it treated my mother.

When they suggested I leave both my job and my husband, I couldn't face it. I was terrified of finding myself, back where I had come from. Unfortunately, I could not manage to live like I was, either. I returned to using drugs, and the counselor I was seeing dropped me. I was given a group I could attend, and I did for a year and a half, but I did little here either. I would have had to be honest and admit my life was out of control and I needed to do something drastic to change it. It would take another six years before I reached a level of despair severe enough to push me to take the action that I needed to take.

On June 11, 1992, I was admitted into a stabilization unit

and then to residential treatment. At 8:30 that morning I staggered, still intoxicated, down the halls of the institution where I would begin to make the most drastic change in my entire life.

Getting there had not been easy. I had to reach the point where I could not stand it anymore, the point where I had considered that death had become a better solution than living the way I was living.

My marriage had reached an impasse, and there was nothing left to save. Staying any longer was only a slow form of torture for both of us. I had become careless with my life. I no longer cared how much I used or how many different things I used at the same time. I had begun to see an addiction doctor, and the same suggestion of residential treatment was on the table.

Finally, it seemed like a better idea than staying in the living hell I was living. I agreed, and very quickly the bed became available. I thought I would take a break from my life and then maybe I could figure out what to do.

I never thought that I would change my entire life. I never thought I would take the steps that were suggested to me six years prior. Treatment would change everything. It would be the hardest journey I would ever take because I would have to review all that had happened, in order to understand how I had got to where I found myself, and to realize that I could change myself.

It would be the first time that I had stopped to grieve all that I had lost, and all that addiction had taken from me. I had remained numb for twenty-one years of my life, and I had run from all the hurt I had experienced in the thirty-four years of my life. I can't begin to explain how painful that process was, how lost I remained, and for how long before I would emerge from this. It would take seventeen years before I could walk without the desire to kill myself raging in my mind when I wasn't busy.

Work would allow me to survive, because in helping others, I found a way to survive my own painful journey.

PART TWO:

RECOVERY

I am going to talk about the recovery business in Ottawa. I am not going to name any of the places that I will talk about because I don't think the names really matter. What I want to tell you about is how the business of treatment was handled and funding had everything to do with that. The attitude towards addiction also played a huge part.

I completed a twenty-eight-day residential treatment program in 1992. It was a time when addiction was not looked upon very favorably. People with addiction had to be transformed from the unhealthy people they were into something that could be worked with.

It was a tear you down and build you back up approach. In essence they needed to break you, then once broken they could build you back up. What that translated to is they could be confronting and if you weren't looking like you were going to be successful, they could give you the boot.

This was directly related to funding. Your statistics mattered. If you were serving people, and they weren't succeeding in getting well, and staying well, then you weren't providing the treatment that would be funded. Statistics mattered.

At the treatment center where I attended, they had two and a half pages of rules that you couldn't break. They had a three-strike rule, break three rules and they could kick you out. As I watched what was going on in stabilization, it seemed like they were waiting until it looked like people could function and participate before they were sent to the treatment center. At the treatment center, you had to be able to do what was expected of you. If it looked like you weren't functioning, you got kicked out.

Some people got kicked out who were just not taking things seriously. If you got caught in a relationship with someone in treatment with you, they kicked you out. I also saw people get kicked out who were obviously very traumatized and shut down. They weren't going to make it through the program. Those who got kicked out were not included in the treatment center's statistics. Only those who completed the program were included in the stats. I believe that the way that the treatment centers were being funded had a lot to do with what they were doing. If you are funded for your success, then you better make sure that you don't gamble on anyone who looks like they're not going to make it.

I saw a couple of incidents when I was in treatment at this hospital that stayed with me. One was a young woman who was in the detox with me and rarely spoke. She looked very shell-shocked. It was clear that there was something that had haunted her. She had a scar that ran down one side of her face, and she was a small person that often reminded me of a child. It wasn't until we were both at the treatment center that I finally heard her speak.

I was in the smoking room one night and she spoke to me. It kind of surprised me because I didn't expect her to speak. She told me what had happened to her that resulted in the scar she had. She said her father had cut her. She had not come from a very safe home, so she left it as soon as she could, which ended up with her living on the street and using drugs.

I never knew why she chose to speak to me that night. I felt very sad for her because she seemed so frightened. She had been in the detox for a very long time before they sent her to treatment because she was so silent. She didn't last long in treatment before they kicked her out.

I remember she showed up for gym, and she had stopped for a smoke outside with a number of other clients who smoked. We were not allowed to do that. She had also forgotten her running shoes. That was enough to strike her out. She already had another rule violation previously. I knew they used the rules to be able to get rid of people they wanted to get rid of because they didn't apply them unless you were someone who wasn't a good bet. She wasn't. She had too much trauma and it was affecting her ability to manage the program. The rules just allowed them to get rid of her without admitting that was the reason. I heard she ended up with AIDS later. I don't believe she survived it.

Another woman I was in detox with was kicked out because she had asked if she could leave temporarily to attend her son's funeral; he had committed suicide while she was on the unit. They told her if she left, she couldn't come back. She left, of course, because she obviously would. She called me some time later, and she was still trying to get some help but was unable to get back into the detox or get other help.

Just to give you a flavor of the interaction in treatment at the time, I was told by my counselor that I was an addict, that I had always been an addict and that I would die an addict. It was all in an effort to confront me with my current state and encourage me to make a different choice, but it was delivered in a way that was confronting.

I'd have to say that I was probably not the most defiant person there, so I'm sure that some conversations could have gotten much more heated. I was successful in treatment, and I completed the twenty-eight days and graduated from the program. I was given weekly follow-ups, followed by monthly sessions that lasted one year. I never relapsed. That is rather unusual, and I can only understand it from the fact that I came in because I was chronically suicidal and going back to using for me would have meant taking my life.

When you think of their stats being the priority it's pretty grim. Here we have an illness that we now know has a relapse rate associated with it, as do many other chronic conditions, and it's stunning that this was taking place. If we were applying this same principle to other chronic illnesses related to the unhealthy behaviors of the patients, hospitals would have been sued. Could you imagine being told that if you have another heart attack related to your unhealthy eating habits, we are not going to treat you? What if your cancer reoccurs and you are still smoking, and the doctors say, "Well, that's it. We are not going to treat your cancer because you are still smoking"?

This was the attitude towards people with addiction at that time. Even though the disease theory suggested that addiction was not a moral failing, that attitude remained in play for a very long time. The idea was that if you were deliberately making yourself ill by your immoral attitude towards alcohol and drugs, you were not going to be extended a great deal of tolerance. I believe that the problem that has existed right up to today is that people don't seem to grasp what the meaning of the concept of addiction is. It has never been adequately defined.

Addiction, by the nature of the word, means that the person cannot stop using on their own, and even when they have been stopped, they are still at risk of returning to use for some time after they stop. Addiction is a state of an overwhelming pull to continue taking the drug or drugs that have become associated with relief from something that feels unbearable. So even if someone stops using it, there is a pull to use again every time the stress level rises enough to trigger the desire for relief. It has become a conditioned behavior from years of repeating it over and over again. This persists, even to the point that when it no longer provides the relief it once did, the person will continue doing it, hoping for the same original relief that they experienced in the beginning and hoping to avoid the withdrawal effects of stopping.

The ACE studies tell us that a common road to addiction is through trying to relieve the effects of trauma. Given this, every time a person stops using, the undealt with trauma resurfaces again, and this triggers the desire to use to eliminate the effects or to numb the pain. The Ace study has given us the best understanding of addiction that we have had. It makes the most sense of addiction and, by its definition, elicits the best response, a compassionate one. It does, however, call for a response. It does see addiction as an inadequate response to trauma, as well as one that can continue to perpetuate trauma. It challenges our current policies on responding to addiction because, in doing so, we are ignoring the trauma. People are addicted because we refuse to provide services to treat trauma or prevent trauma from occurring. In refusing to treat addicted people, we perpetuate addiction because we will not treat their trauma and providing them with drugs is saying that explicitly.

There has been a resistance to understanding the relationship between trauma and addiction and given the often out-of-control behavior exhibited by people active in their addiction, there is no surprise as to why. Addicted people do not seem to be able to engender the same sympathetic response that we see in something like juvenile diabetes, for example. Their behavior makes them unattractive and causes problems for other people.

There are few redeeming qualities to the drunken guy on the bus who is yelling at you for no reason, or the person in a drug-induced psychosis that has incorporated you into their belief that people are staring at them and judging them. It can be more than a little bit problematic.

This is another key issue in addiction that never gets

addressed, and therefore it is hard to gain any traction for responses that might have a better chance of working. What we see is a pendulum swinging back and forth from the haters to those personally impacted by having lost their family members to the disease. One has only to watch videos of the downfall of people like Amy Winehouse or Sid Vicious to see how utterly ugly it can get.

I am often convinced that the series "The Walking Dead" was based on addiction and its effects. It's just that horrific at times. Look at someone who is addicted to methamphetamine, where they have suffered the complete destruction of their face and teeth. I'm sure that people often don't believe that it can look that bad, but I have personally seen people who have completely altered their look after years of meth use. I worked at one of the shelters, and the physical appearance of people who were addicted was frightening. They were often covered in scabs and open wounds. They were like walking bacterial infection.

Another issue that I believe is a key issue and also doesn't get presented on the tables by those trying to improve the way we view addiction, is the reality of the connection between crime and addiction. People, neighborhoods, and businesses are affected by behaviors addicted people engage in, to get the money to buy illegal drugs. We can't just ignore this like it's politically incorrect to talk about it in the same conversation that we talk about our need to support treatment. Not to address it is to say that, for all of the people whose lives have been damaged or affected by the addiction of another person, we don't wish to discuss this. We don't want you bringing this up because it may interfere with what we are trying to do. We don't want to paint people with addiction in a negative way. I'm not sure what fairy tale we should be telling if we choose not to speak the truth, but in doing so, we alienate a huge amount of people.

The fact of the matter is that one person's addiction affects multiple people and aspects of society. One addicted person can cause damage on a very large scale over the course of their active addiction. We cannot ignore this because the symptoms of addiction have dire consequences for other people. This should escalate our efforts to treat it rather than accept it as the choice of one person who is ill, by definition. When we were dealing with COVID, we were willing to go to all lengths to enforce upon people what was expected of them so others were not in danger, yet we allow addicted people to endanger other people's lives with impunity. They were one population who were completely exempt from any restrictions around COVID. I watched them board public transit absolutely cost-free without masks and intoxicated throughout the worst of the pandemic. I ended up contracting COVID as a result of this and no amount of contacting the local transit authorities or politicians did anything to stop this.

After I completed my treatment, it was deemed quite correctly, I believe, that I would not be successful if I went back home to my husband and back to my job. By the last week of treatment, I had made up my mind that I would not do this. My sister offered me the opportunity to move in with her, and the treatment center had suggested a second-stage house that I was willing to go to.

I had to wait about a month before moving in. I was worried once again that I was going to go back to poverty and that the second stage house would be some run-down place like what I had grown up in. Once more I felt myself falling back to that past I so feared ever returning to. The house turned out to be a really nice place in an upscale end of the city. I remember my interview. I thought I was at the director's place and when she told me to pick a room, I was shocked. I'd never lived in such a rich home. I would stay here for almost two years as I tried to get well enough to manage on my own.

These places financed themselves partially by having residents pay rent. I would pay rent there based on a disability I was receiving from my work at that time. I was involved in an investigation into the attack by my boss on me, instigated by my work. When I had refused to return to work, they had threatened me with the police if I did not reveal why, so I was given no choice. I believe this was because of previous embezzlement by another manager. I had left just before they had discovered what he was up to, and they may have thought that I knew something about it. They may have thought something similar was taking place.

The investigation took a year, and they found in my favor which meant very little. They paid me back my holiday entitlement. They had the manager off with full pay for the entire time, and he returned to work. I was given two years long term disability until I told them to just stop the disability because I was done. By that point I had been hired by the treatment center associated with the second stage house where I had been living.

When I entered this aspect of the addiction treatment world, these places often employed people who had recovered from addiction themselves. They might have some level of education related to psychology, counseling, or addiction, but there would be many who were simply people who had been successful in their recovery. They were often longer-term residential treatment places, and they often had second-stage houses attached to them. There were also outpatient addiction treatment centers as well. There were some addiction-related counselors working separately and some counseling-related centers that worked with addiction and other related issues. I had contact with a number of these agencies, and I would like to describe some of the experiences I had in these places. I hope that outlining some of the experiences I had will also give you an idea of how addiction was being approached at the time. I believe that this reflects the lack of investment in addressing addiction as an illness.

The second stage house I lived in had eight residents at any one time. We all paid rent based on income but, for the most part, people were on Ontario works which was for those who had not been working at all, unless they had other insurance coverage. The residents came from a number of different sources. It was initially staffed twenty-four hours a day by three counselors. Two counselors had lived experience as a qualification and were responsible for watching that things went well and that there was someone to whom the clients could speak. They worked the evening and overnight shifts. The third counselor worked during the day and had an educational background.

When I first arrived, there wasn't much going on at the house in the area of counseling or programming. It was a new place that had just opened. I took advantage of what was available in the community and applied for support through an outpatient addiction service. I saw a counselor who dealt with adult child issues in a separate place since I had been very negatively affected by growing up in an addicted home, and this had been identified in treatment as a significant issue for me. I paid for that counseling on a sliding fee scale. I was receiving long term disability from my work at the time. The outpatient service was at no cost to me and provided a counselor and two groups a week. I chose to access these services because I had been very destabilized from coming off the years of substance abuse.

I remember watching a film while at residential treatment called "The Heart of a Child." I was traumatized by seeing that film. It was the story of three children living in a home where there was parental addiction. It showed how each child had responded differently to the addictive behaviors of the parents. I felt a sense of panic as I watched the movie because I didn't know how they knew about what had gone on in my house and how they managed to make a movie out of it. I could barely watch it, yet I couldn't look away because I was shocked. It was like being confronted with a horrible thing that you had barely managed to survive and had kept at a distance from you all of your life because you knew you couldn't possibly deal with it.

I sobbed when I saw that movie. I saw myself, the lost child, standing in the midst of absolute chaos and pain. All the tears I wasn't allowed to cry began to pour out of me. I felt devastated and broken. I was reduced to that kid again, trying to become invisible so no one would come near me.

They had a psychodrama exercise afterwards where you created a living sculpture of your family and placed yourself in it. I could not manage anything at that point. I thought about it and all I could think was I would just walk outside because that's where I had been in my family. What I really tried to do was melt through my chair. I couldn't open my eyes or speak, and they just left me alone. I think they could also see that I couldn't handle this, so they didn't push me to participate.

This reaction and all the codependent behaviors I had developed in relation to my mother, and those that showed up in treatment, made it obvious that I needed to get help, or I would not be able to recover from my addiction. I listened to the advice I was given, and I set about trying to recover.

I also attended twelve-step meetings regularly and eventually I also attended adult child meetings as well. I grabbed onto anything I could find that would help me because I knew that for me failure would mean death because if I didn't make it in recovery, I was going to kill myself. I had made a firm commitment that I could not go back to where I had been because there was nothing to go back to. I had reached the place in my use where nothing relieved the pain I was experiencing, and that pain had become intolerable. In treatment, that pain still existed and became more acute as the reality of the life I had lived up to that point began to return to me in memories, nightmares, and extreme emotions.

At some point at the residence where I was living, it became apparent that I was rarely there, and I was asked to meet with the day counselor there just to check in and see what I was up to.

It's important to point out how vulnerable you are when you have come out of an extremely dysfunctional home and have been numbing yourself for over twenty years and, as a result, know almost nothing of who you are or how you got that way.

I had never been mothered. I was a deeply wounded kid who had to become an adult because my mother demanded it. I'd spent a lifetime trying to prove I was worth my existence in any place I found myself. I had to do everything that was expected of me. My mother had given me the message that she could not have me being any sort of a problem because she had to deal with my sister, who was acting out constantly. I had to require nothing of my mother and, more than that, I had to offer up everything in order to be allowed to stay. This is the kind of stuff that gets played out everywhere in your life until you find a way to learn to be different.

When I was in residential treatment, I developed a huge sense of neediness towards my counselor there. Even her harsh words about my addiction didn't shift this because, after all, my mother had not been a kind person towards me, and I loved her immensely. I also saw for the first time there that I had a very strange way of responding to the person I perceived in a mother-like role. I would not ask to speak to her even if I really needed to. I stayed away and, for the most part, acted like I didn't need her help at all. At one point she asked me if I wanted a new counselor, and I was very quick to respond that I didn't want a new counselor. I was mortified that she would just drop me. It really rocked me because I had this huge drive towards wanting to be with her. I had to ask myself what the hell my behavior was about. What the hell was I doing? At some level I realized that this was exactly what I had done with my mother. She had made it clear to me that she had enough trouble parenting my brother and sister, so she didn't need me to make things any more difficult for her. I was doing the same thing with my counselor. I wasn't her only client and so I'd better not exacerbate her, or she would kick me to the curb. This was all the more reason I couldn't understand her asking me if I wanted a different counselor.

It would also be important to mention that for the first week after I arrived at residential treatment, I had no counselor assigned to me. The counselor that was to be assigned to me was on holiday. Other than attending groups, I was left to my own devices because homework was assigned by your counselor. I read just about every book I could find in the place and, as a result, the first time I met with my counselor I announced that I was shocked to discover I was in denial. She made it clear that she would be the person to say I was in denial and not me. I was banned from reading any more during my treatment. This was just an unfortunate event that I was left alone in treatment for a week, but it was probably one of the worst things you can do to a kid who has been abandoned since birth. Left alone and without instruction, I did what I had done as a child. I looked in books for the answers.

This tendency to distance myself while feeling terribly needy, which I developed in my relationship with my mother, would play out many times over and over. It was about to get played out again in the second stage house with the day counselor. It would grow over the two-year period that I stayed there until it felt as painful as the original place where it developed.

This is the consequence of growing up in dysfunction. Instead of having relationships with your family that are nurturing and growth-inspiring, you end up in terrible binds that leave you playing the same losing hand over and over. In my home I could not ask my mother to love me or to hold me because she was already overwhelmed. I had to step out of the way, but I still needed her desperately. Because she had alienated me from my peers through her neglect and her demand that I do whatever she needed me to do whenever she needed me to do it, I had no way of making up for her lack of love. The few friends I ever had were not there for any length of time, and I would be alone again. I learned to yearn for her love from a distance while the pain inside just grew. I spent hours alone experiencing that pain, and this would get played out again in the second stage house.

When I met the counselor, I was cautious, but I liked her almost from the first day. She seemed like a motherly person, and she had kids of her own. She was not old enough to be my mother but more like a friend. The unmet infancy needs in me responded to her and I had no way to stop this from happening, first because initially I didn't know it and second because the need in me was so great there was little that would have stopped it.

I would only come to realize it when it was too late, and I had developed a dysfunctional attachment to her. If someone had diagnosed this, they would have said that I had borderline personality disorder. My unhealthy relationship with my mother meant that my relationships would be unstable and characterized by extreme emotions. In my marriage, I had certainly demonstrated some pretty extreme reactions to my husband that swung from care to absolute rage and hatred. If you added a bit of alcohol to that situation it would be catastrophic for him. The constant suicidal ideation was also a symptom of BPD. Unfortunately, that diagnosis usually translates to people you never want to have to work with. I don't believe I was ever formally diagnosed with it, but one doctor I saw certainly was leaning toward that conclusion after a suicide attempt.

This is where some of the problems in treatment can be found. People with long term addiction have usually found their way there through an inability to function in the world successfully, and so they tend to turn to substances or behaviors to mitigate the unresolved emotions and the fallout of having been raised in dysfunctional homes. Many may never get help, and they, in turn, will negatively affect their children or other family members around them. It's the gift that keeps on giving.

I chose at a rather young age not to have any children because I couldn't bear to damage them in the way that I had been, and I didn't believe that I could avoid doing so. Both my sister and my brother had children, and they seemed to have turned out fine for the most part. I feel that I was damaged in a way that would not have made this possible. In my life I have never felt truly loved by anyone, at least not in the way that a mother loves her child. I don't believe that I would have treated a child like they were the ones that needed to be loved. The hole in me was too big.

The counselor that I became attached to had her own undealt with issues as well. She had three children, all from different fathers, and one was still an infant. She had her own history of addiction. She had her own history of dysfunctional relationships with her parents, and she had chosen partners who also had their own issues.

I first realized there was a problem for me when I became aware of an overwhelming need to be near her. At times it was enough to just be somewhere where I could see her. She was the mother now of eight highly unhealthy people. At some level I understood this, and I began to just stay somewhere in the vicinity of her. This need grew and grew over time. Eventually, when she left for the day, I was beside myself, and I would stay in my room and try to bear the pain it brought about.

I had also reduced the activities I had outside of the house just to be near her. My emotions became very erratic around this time, and I would cry uncontrollably for hours on end. This then shifted to uncontrolled heights, followed by crashes that went on for days. I felt like I was losing my mind. The staff met with the director to discuss the clients, and it was decided that I would have to see a psychiatrist because there was obviously something wrong with me. They made the appointment for me.

I have seen a lot of questionable behavior from professionals over time since I came into recovery and since working in the addiction field. This was one of those times when you have to ask yourself where these people get their training. I arrived at the appointment, and I was very nervous about it because the idea that there was something wrong with my head harkened back to the accusations my mother had made about me as a kid. Was she finally going to be proven right?

The psychiatrist was a young man working out of a mental health hospital. He asked me why I had come to see him, and I explained that the place where I lived made the appointment because I was thinking about taking my life, and I had been having difficulty with my emotions. He said that he didn't know why the house I lived at had made the appointment because he did not want to see anybody from their place. I was feeling barely controlled rage, and he asked me why I was so angry. I told him that I hated "fucking" psychiatrists, and that was it, appointment over. I couldn't believe that they had sent me to this guy and his only response had been that he didn't want to see anybody from the place where I was living. It was difficult enough for me to have to go to the appointment but then to have this guy just reject me because of the place where I was living was too much for me at that moment. I couldn't manage it. I wasn't well enough to handle that.

When I went back to the house, they were insistent that I needed to see a psychiatrist, and so they made another appointment with the same guy. I told them that he had said he did not want to see me, but they made it a condition of my staying there, so I had to go back. I went back to him again. He said he did not want to see me or anyone else from the house where I lived. I told him that maybe he should have this out with the staff there rather than take it out on me. I felt completely helpless in this situation. I felt like some sort of rejected ping pong ball. Emotionally I was already a mess, so I did not need this. My whole life I had felt like I did not matter, and my life was worth nothing, and here I was in the office of a person who was supposed to help people, and he clearly didn't even want me there.

I hope that anyone reading this also thinks this is improper because I cannot, in retrospect, understand how a professional could treat a person seeking help in such a way. If he had an issue with this recovery house, why not call them up and tell them that he did not want to treat clients from their facility? Why would he choose to take this out on the person who had been sent there by the facility? I was the person suffering from a mental health issue, but he thought it was OK for him to blame me for the facility sending me there to see him. Let's not forget the fact that I had disclosed that I was suicidal.

He would not be the last professional I would see acting in ways that really made me wonder about how this kind of thing goes on and on, and nothing is done about it. I am writing this book to bring some of this to light. I could choose to name the individuals involved, but that would gain nothing. There have been numerous times that I have tried to directly address the unethical behavior of professionals, but they are so protected that they can act in ways that directly lead to the deaths of people, and nothing can be done.

I am hoping that as I document these unethical behaviors you will come to see that it is a problem that needs to seriously be addressed. I was seriously suicidal, and this man was more interested in his spiteful attitude towards the center that housed me, than in doing anything to help me.

He is not the first psychiatrist that I have seen act in ways that amount to the complete disregard of the lives of the people who are looking to them for help. Some of those people have died, unfortunately. The dysfunction in the system exists at all levels. The lives of those who died were not deemed important enough to have attracted any attention. Their loved ones lacked the power to fight against those who had not seen their lives as significant enough to be worth the help they could have provided.

I was eventually referred to another psychiatrist who agreed to see me. I was put on medication when he explained he couldn't work with me because I was so unwell that I needed something to help me with my emotional state. This was hard for me to accept because I didn't want to have to take medication, but I would have to accept it because I couldn't function the way I was. I was by then over a year abstinent from drugs, and my mental state had become worse than when I had been using drugs. I often said I felt more normal when I had been drinking and using drugs than I now felt not using anything. I would come to understand that I had been self-medicating. Eventually I would find out that I had Bipolar 2 Disorder. My mother's sister had it, and my mother showed symptoms of it as well. I might not have ever gotten this disorder, but the years of smoking pot had made the chances much higher.

This would be the beginning of the years of changing medications, until the final combination was found that worked. I had a huge difficulty talking to this man, and the experience often left me in a state of rage. At one point, in response to my talking about suicide, he told me that one patient he saw almost cut off his hand in his office while trying to slit his wrist, and another had stuck himself to the floor while trying the same thing. I don't know about you, but I failed to see the therapeutic benefit of telling me those stories, whether true or not.

I had been seeing him for six months before I decided that he was not helping me at all. It was about the time when I was moving out of the second stage house, and I would choose to go on to find another doctor to see. The psychiatrist I left was eventually charged with sexually abusing one of his patients. I would later find out that this was also something that was common.

The situation with the counselor at the house changed over time until I realized that we had become friends, and I had become her confidant. This was an exact repeat of what had happened in my relationship with my mother. I had become my mother's partner and confidant.

The Counselor began to tell me her story and with what she was currently dealing. She was still connected to her young son's dad, who was actively using drugs, and she was in a lot of distress about this. She told me about her parents and her other children. I went to her place a few times. She was angry about how she had been treated when her son was born because they had made accusations about her drug use and health issues with her baby. She said she would like to start an underground group that could care for addicted women's babies when they went to treatment so that they would not have to deal with Social Services and their condemnation.

This was becoming increasingly more painful for me. I

tried to tell her at one point that I had transference issues with her and that I believed that she also had countertransference with me. I have always been a very keen learner. I had returned to university, and I had been taking psychology courses, so I had been learning about this, and again it was making sense to me. She dismissed my concerns and obviously did not get the point that this was causing me a lot of pain. This was what had happened to me with my mother, and my transference with her was like the issue I had with my mother.

She asked me once if she could put something she wanted to buy on my credit card, and she would pay me back. I did not know that this was an unethical thing for her to do, and I let her use my credit card. She paid a portion of the money back, but she never paid the full amount. This was not the last unethical behavior I would see from her, but it would come later when I had left the house.

After I moved out, she kept calling me, and I was really experiencing the pain around my abandonment with my mother. It had been stirred up quite a bit while I was living at the second stage house. At one point I had to ask her again to stop calling me because it was not helping with my mental state. My greatest wound was the relationship I had with my mother. It was the most painful experience of my life. I had not recovered from it, and it would be a long time before I would. This counselor had wounded me in precisely the same place, and I could not get her to understand that she was continuing to hurt me, and I could not manage it.

I believe countertransference is one of the very real dangers that cropped up over and over in this field. It was the fact that many people who worked in it had their own often unhealed histories, and that made countertransference a serious risk if it was not acknowledged and worked through. Countertransference happens and that is not the issue. It is the unwillingness to acknowledge that it is taking place that causes the problem. This is where supervision or doing one's own therapy work can help. If you are in therapy yourself, you can bring this up in therapy and work through it, so you do not act it out on the client. In supervision you talk about your clients and where you are struggling with them, and counter-transference can be explored.

Relapse Prevention

While I was living at the second stage house, I was very unstable in the first seven months of my recovery. I had severe Post-Acute Withdrawal Symptoms, and they were causing serious issues for me. I was going through an investigation into what had happened to me at the bank where I had worked and where the manager had sexually assaulted me. When I told them what had happened, they decided to launch an investigation. This meant that an investigator would be meeting with me regularly.

Their head office was not in Ottawa, so the person had to come to Ottawa. I first received a call from him asking that I meet him in his room at his hotel. I was astounded that he would be asking this since the complaint was about a sexual assault, so why was he asking me to meet him, a man I did not know, in his hotel room? This made me think they were trying to discredit my character by making it seem that I was the kind of woman who was accustomed to meeting men I didn't know in hotels. I felt offended and angry that this was how they were approaching this.

I called head office and told them that the investigator would have to meet me at the house in the presence of a union representative. All this had really been difficult for me because there were things the manager was asking and a lot of questions that they were asking me. They knew I was in treatment for substance addiction. They claimed they didn't know that the manager had alcohol problems. I knew that they did because he had gone to head office for some training, and I went up there just after he did and all I heard were the stories of how much he was drinking while he was there.

The effect this was having on my mental health was not good, and my Post-Acute Withdrawal Symptoms became increasingly worse. At this point, I was asked if I would be willing to go into Relapse Prevention treatment at the men's treatment center associated with the house. I agreed to this because I could not achieve any stability emotionally, and the Post-Acute Withdrawal Symptoms were also very pronounced.

Terrence Gorski's Staying Sober Book

Post-Acute Withdrawal Symptoms: these are symptoms that occur after you have finished physical withdrawal. They consist of six symptoms, including:

1. **Memory Problems:** short term memory is affected, so you can't remember something someone said ten minutes ago. You can also have some temporary long-term memory loss where you can't remember significant events from the past.
2. **Sleep Problems:** you can't fall asleep easily, you can't stay asleep, you find yourself falling asleep during the day, you sleep at odd times of the day, you have disturbing dreams, and when you do sleep, you sometimes sleep for very long periods.
3. **Problems with Thinking:** you have repetitive thoughts, negative thought patterns, circular thinking, difficulty with abstract concepts, rumination, errors in thinking.
4. **Problems with emotions:** severe highs and lows, emotional overreactions, emotional numbness, and inability to understand or identify one's feelings.

5. **Accident Proneness:** loss of balance, difficulty judging space and height, clumsiness, knocking things over, dizziness or lack of balance.
6. **Difficulties managing stress:** overreact to small stresses, no reaction to big stresses, stress aggravates all the other symptoms, making them worse.

These symptoms occur as the brain is trying to return to normal after having altered itself to deactivate the effects of the drug. This is the phenomenon of tolerance. The brain is always seeking homeostasis for optimum survival. If the brain senses that something is not functioning properly, it will make alterations to return the system to a balanced state, as it does in response to a drug that is causing issues that may cause survival risks. For example, when you drink too much, you become off balance, but when tolerance develops, this is when the brain makes alterations that correct the balance problems and then more alcohol will be required to cause the imbalance to happen again. The brain is deactivating the effect of alcohol to enhance survival. It recognizes that the effects of alcohol are threatening survival. It does this with all drugs of abuse. A regular drinker can drink more without appearing as intoxicated as someone who only drinks occasionally. When the addicted person stops their use, the system is still in an altered state related to using a substance regularly. The brain is altered to compensate for the effects of the presence of the drug. Without the presence of the drug, the system is now off balance because it is correcting something that's not there. It will take time for this to be corrected and for the brain to go back to normal. Until then, the person experiences the symptoms of Post-Acute Withdrawal. Recovery from this is estimated to be about eighteen months, and the severity of the symptoms varies from person to person, depending on the damage done to the brain.

Recovery Basics are a set of activities and behaviors that help heal and feed the brain so it can heal faster. These things include good nutrition, relaxation, meditation, exercise, sleep, therapy, recreation, stress reduction skills and learning problem-solving skills, and all go a long way to helping this process. Stress will increase the symptoms and throw the person off balance. Unfortunately, if the person uses, the symptoms will disappear temporarily. The symptoms can also be severe enough that a person can feel like they are going crazy.

At the time that Relapse Prevention was suggested to me, I was having serious difficulties managing stress due to the investigation with the bank and all of the memories it was bringing up for me. I thought I could just walk away from the bank and not go back, and suddenly I was stuck in the middle of an investigation I had not wanted to initiate. I was so stressed out that I was becoming dysfunctional. I couldn't make it through a doorway without running into the door frame. I couldn't stand on the bus because I had no balance. My emotions were already a problem, and the investigation just made that worse. My sleep was terrible. I found that I couldn't sleep with the light off, something that had not been a problem since I was a kid. I was having serious nightmares, and when I woke up from them, I had a hard time going back to sleep. I could see I was in danger.

I had a lot of cravings to use, and I couldn't understand it because I was doing everything I had been told to do. I felt like I was somehow a failure at recovery because I wasn't getting better; I was getting worse. When it was suggested that I go through the treatment program for Relapse Prevention, I figured it couldn't hurt and maybe it would help me.

It had one strange twist. It was a men's treatment program, and they had never had a woman there. I figured I could handle that because I often related better to men than to women. I had been a tomboy as a kid, and I had never understood women since I was never given a chance to be a female growing up. It was five days a week for three months. I would go there every day and come home afterwards, while the guys were living there. It was the best thing I did for myself.

This program was based on Terence Gorski's Staying Sober workbook and book. It was intensive and involved a lot of homework. I believe I learned a lot about myself and my addiction in that treatment program. It was destabilizing at times because it brought out the Post-Acute Withdrawal Symptoms more, but it also explained them, so I finally didn't feel like I was crazy. I went through it with six guys, and we got to know each other well during those three months.

I really appreciated what I learned, and I soaked it up like a sponge. I have always had this habit of both participating and observing at the same time. The woman who was the director of the center was leading the group, and I learned so much from her. She was a skilled counselor with great insight and a great ability to cut through the crap. I also really appreciated the material in the text and workbook and the videos we watched. I learned so much from Terence Gorski's work that I became a great advocate of this program. I felt like it had saved my life at that point. I could see the process that it took you through and I could see how and why it worked. I thought it had real merit.

Not long after I completed the program, the director came to me and asked me if I would like to try working as a volunteer in the Relapse Prevention program at the center. I was both surprised and excited to be given this opportunity and so I said yes. I had a good analytical mind and that I had really understood the program and that's why she offered me a chance to try it. I was still living at the second stage house that was associated with this treatment center.

Was it ethical? Should they have asked a client to work

in the treatment center? This is questionable, but it wasn't that uncommon at the time. This was the state of addiction treatment. Beggars couldn't be choosers. It's not like anybody really wanted to work with addicts at that point. It was 1994.

Back at the second stage house the lines began to blur there as well. Suddenly there was no overnight staff, and I was being asked to keep an eye on things. That was a bigger problem for me. I was back to taking over my mother's job. All the while I was struggling with my own mental health and feeling like I was reliving one of my biggest traumas. I had developed the behavior of cutting and that had become a problem for me. I was too ashamed to talk to anyone about it because it didn't make any sense to me. I found myself balancing between my precarious mental health and my ability to act like there was nothing wrong and attend to whatever tasks I was expected to do.

I also vacillated between infancy and rebellious adolescence in the second stage house. Some of my behaviors were downright juvenile, as if I was trying to have the adolescence I never had. All this was hard to make sense of and, looking back, I see that it was the stages of childhood that I was never allowed to have, but they disappeared when, once again, I took on the role of pseudo-parent in another dysfunctional family. I think it is amazing that we repeat our history over and over as if there is no other history that we were ever meant to have.

Even in my real family at the time, my sister was asking for my help while her own marriage fell apart, and my father was in active addiction, with everyone expecting that I should know how to fix it. My whole family had a huge shift at the same time as my entry into recovery. All of our marriages ended in the same year. A year later we would all lose our long-term jobs. I figured we were just a family that liked to disintegrate together.

My father re-entered my life after my mother's death. My

sister had found him and had been going to see him prior to my mother's death, and I had chosen not to see him then. When I had contact with him, he was drinking but hiding this from his family and my sister. He began contacting me. I was actively addicted at the time, and I didn't understand what he wanted from me. He would call me from hotel rooms where he was drunk. In my early recovery he was drinking again, and I found it very triggering to be around him. He had been actively alcoholic when we were little kids, and there had been many physical fights between him and my mother, and I think feelings from this part of my childhood were being triggered by his being under the influence.

I called him to the second stage house where I was at the time and told him that he had every right to drink and that this was none of my business. I explained that I could not be around him because I was trying to leave that behind. I told him if he ever changed his mind and decided to stop drinking, I would like to have a relationship with him. He went to detox two weeks later and then to treatment. He stayed in recovery until he died and became a very liked and respected person in the recovery community in Brockville. He never rose to the occasion to be a father to me. I don't think he could, and I don't think I could allow him to be that. I think I represented what he wanted to leave behind: the guilt of having abandoned his children. I was there for him when he was dying. I told him I loved him as I held his hand. I believe I did for him what he could never do for me. I think all I ever wanted was for him to say he was sorry. It was his leaving that caused us so much pain and difficulty. He went on to have another life, and he had comforts that we never knew. He never left us anything. The least that he could have done was to say that he was sorry. It wasn't much to ask.

My First Job in the Addiction Field

I began my journey into the field of addiction when I was asked to volunteer to work at the men's treatment center connected to the second stage house I was living at. At first, I just did some research and a presentation to the staff. I was finally asked to start learning how to deliver the Relapse Prevention program. I started the first day sitting in with the house manager. Someone came down to say that he had a phone call. He left and never came back.

From that point forward, I worked in the Relapse Prevention Program with clients on my own. It would be important to point out how unprofessional it was for this place to simply leave me running a group with no supervision from day one.

I applied what I had always applied in my life. I stood up to the challenge and did what was asked of me. It would be important to say that I was an intelligent person with strong academic skills. It had been recommended that I pursue an academic education when I was in grade school because I was very bright. I chose to go to an art course in high school because I had grown to love drawing, and I wanted to be an artist. My mother wanted me to go to university or college, but of course she couldn't help with that, but she often said that when she died there would be some money from insurance that could help. She had an educational insurance policy for the three of us but said we could only have it if we went to school. When she died, I went to college for Fine Arts.

Even during my active use I was attending university

in a BA program in Anthropology and getting good marks, so I think there was some reason for why I was asked to do this work. I had always tried to figure out why people did the things they did, and from a young age I had an acute ability to understand what a person was feeling. This is often an offshoot of growing up in an alcoholic family. You must be good at reading others and sensing the tension in a room if you are going to have any chance of survival.

Reading had also been a pastime for a kid who had no friends and spent so much time alone. I think it was part of what alienated me from my family so much. I thought very differently than they did because I was exposing myself to knowledge and ideas that they had no knowledge of. I was always trying to figure out the world I was living in. Why did one people hate another? Why were people treated differently because of the color of their skin or their nationality? Why would one person hurt another? Why did some people kill?

Being alienated from my peer group also affected me. I did my homework because what else was there to do? Being a victim of neglect directly impacted the way others responded to me and this left me alone and ashamed. I was often dressed in dirty and worn clothing, with unwashed hair, unbrushed teeth, and I smelled from a lack of regular bathing.

I developed a fascination for a group of people that I thought I could identify with and that became a reading passion throughout my life. I identified with Black Americans. They were being discriminated against because of how they looked, and that resonated with me. I was a child alone in the world, searching for some way to make some sense of where I found myself. It was a very simple connection for a child.

I was twelve years old when I read Eldridge Cleaver's book "Soul on Ice." The righteousness of their fight carried me through many years of complete despair. They became my heroes. I was rooting for them. I was watching them, and I felt hope in their fight and agony at their horrible treatment. Looking back, it must have looked very strange to my family, where my mother certainly expressed some level of bigotry. More than once, she said that she had no idea where I got my thinking, and she wondered whose kid I was. In reality, I was no one's kid. I say all this to explain the kind of adaptation to life that I had. It made me uniquely able to slip into the position of counselor because I had been one since my early childhood.

I had resolved more than one dispute in my family by being the mediator. When my mother discovered that my sister had been going to see her father, a huge angry rift began between them. If their yelling at each other was painful, the angry silence was much worse. I finally realized I had to do something about it. I went to my mother and explained to her how growing up without a father was difficult, because other kids talked about their dads, and we couldn't. I said that there was always curiosity about who he was and what he was doing. I said my sister just wanted to know her dad. She hadn't done this to hurt her; she just really needed to know her dad.

I then went to my sister and explained to her that mom just felt like she had turned away from her and chosen her dad over her. I said she had raised us, and it had been hard, because she had to work every day and she didn't make much money, yet still she chose to keep us and raise us. She felt betrayed by my sister, even though my sister had not done it as an act of betrayal, it had felt that way to my mom. The fight ended. I did this type of thing many times in my family, even between adults who were angry at each other. I had been in training for a long time. Still, this does not make up for the questionable behavior of people who somehow thought I could just step into a counseling position because I had some natural traits.

When you look at the Addiction Field at that time, it wouldn't have seemed that odd that they would have given a person in recovery a job in addiction counseling. Who else would want the job? Even at the residential treatment center where I had first gone for treatment, the staff were either recovering addicts or family members of people with addiction. The Doctor was even a person in recovery since addiction knows no boundaries. I believe that at the time there was so little investment in treating addiction that this was just how it developed.

The rates of pay were and always have been very low. It was an illness that everyone hated. Addicted people were seen as morally low on the ladder because they couldn't just use socially. They had to become lushes who used until they became an utter nuisance. The disease concept had been raised, but few people were willing to accept that as the reason. People were able to control themselves, and addicts just chose not to. The treatment centers also carried that type of belief.

I remember I was sitting in a medical lecture in residential treatment with one of the doctors who was not an addict, who was giving us the explanation of why people became addicted. He was using a study from a rat model. He made a point to say that they had to force the rat to drink alcohol initially, because he wasn't as stupid as we were. We were treated as dishonest, weak-willed, deceptive, and manipulating people who had to be shamed into getting well.

We were also reminded that if we didn't want to be there, no problem; there was a long line of people who wanted to get in. I watched the revolving door of people who left or were kicked out of treatment. I remember being terrified the whole time I was there that they were going to kick me out. If you were called to meet with that doctor, chances were, they were going to kick you out.

He called me to see him once and I thought that this was it. I was done. He explained to me that I wasn't sharing much in the group and that this needed to change. It was easy to see that I had a huge amount of emotion just sitting under the surface, but I had no idea how I was supposed to share that. It's not like I had ever had a lesson in how to talk about what was going on with me. That had never been important in my life. I had never been important in my life.

The rules in the family I grew up in were that you were not to talk about anything and the price for talking was very serious. I was also told I had a secret I was not sharing, and if I did it was a secret to me as well. Nonetheless, I was just supposed to figure that out. Back to my childhood, just do it. Thankfully the film I watched on the addicted family opened the flood gates and satisfied the criteria.

I think this is a problem that all people who have never had any sort of treatment or therapy face. They honestly don't know what to talk about. They have been taught to shut everything down and ignore it all. It took me years to realize all of what had been really going on for me. Some of the most serious things did not surface for the longest time, and when they did, I was shocked that I had not spoken about them.

As an untrained counselor, I used my ability to ask the right questions and gather the information I needed to understand the clients I worked with. I always looked for the story. The workbook asked questions to provide the information I needed to piece together what had happened in each of their lives, which had led to their addiction. We would go over each question in the group, and I would probe further with each response they gave, all the while taking notes that would flesh out the story of their lives. I could be very compassionate. I think all those years of looking at and trying to find out why people did the things that they did worked in my favor.

I had come to understand that there was always a story behind what we do. There are our interpretations of our experiences and our emotional responses to those interpretations.

It didn't matter to the person what the real truth was, because they were busy responding to their own interpretation, and their previous lived experiences were the filter that this interpretation was colored by. I had become aware of this in my family very early in my life.

I cared about the clients. I wanted them to be successful. I wanted them to make it, and I believe, in some way, this was about me wanting to make it as well. I could always find a way to connect to them, and if there were other issues, like mental illness, I tried tirelessly to find them that help.

I decided while I was there that we should find out which psychiatrists in the city would be willing to work with our clients. None of this had been done by the center. We were seeing quite a bit of mental health issues, and many clients would need some medication if they were going to be able to be successful. It was hard to find a psychiatrist who wanted to work with someone with an addiction. The belief at the time was that you had to be free from active use for a minimum of a year or more before a mental health issue could be diagnosed.

Certainly, Post-Acute Withdrawal Symptoms could look a lot like a mental health issue. The problem was if you left a serious mental health issue untreated, the person often couldn't benefit from addiction treatment that often relied on CBT methods. I took it upon myself to mail a letter out to every psychiatrist in the Yellow Pages who treated the adult population to see if they would take referrals for our clients. There were pages of them. I believe that I mailed out letters to at least 150 doctors. Three people responded that they would consider this. I also followed each letter up with a phone call to make sure that I reached every doctor. One of these doctors eventually became involved in our center and offered some individual assessments and a group. I was always looking for ways to improve the services we offered.

The other difficulty with psychiatrists was how you had to

speak to them or write to them. If I suspected that an individual had a mental illness, I had to act like I had no idea of what was going on and give a detailed accounting of the symptoms in the hope the doctor would agree to see the client. In one case I was convinced that a client had hypomanic symptoms and, try as I might, I couldn't get him in to see a doctor. We were unable to work with him because his behavior was so off, and he was unable to gain anything from the treatment. He was finally seen two weeks before he would be leaving, and he was diagnosed with hypomania. Once he was on medication, he was a totally different person. Unfortunately, this did not come in time for him to benefit from treatment. These kinds of issues would plague work in the addiction field for years.

You could not develop a working relationship between the mental health agencies and the addiction agencies because the mental health agencies viewed addiction agencies as agencies that had zero understanding of mental health and would not dialogue with them at all. This went on forever, and even when the terms Addiction and Mental Health were strung together, this did nothing to remedy this problem. I would come to see that the government and other agencies became good at using words to give the illusion that something was taking place when it was not.

I would become aware of the power of words. Words could be used to change the face of the work we did. They could make things disappear that had not, in fact, disappeared at all. Words could be used to remove helping people with addiction completely; in fact, they could make addiction seem to disappear, although, in reality, it continued along its ugly path behind the invisible shield erected to hide it. Words became dangerous in the wrong hands of those in power. I will show how this revealed itself later on.

The other thing that I created while at the men's treatment center was a more comprehensive discharge plan. People would come in having already completed seven or more treatment programs. I couldn't understand what the point was since by now they must know the information on how to prevent a relapse to the point where they could teach it. They were obviously not following through on recommendations. This meant we were wasting our time.

In the discharge plan I made sure that all areas of healthy living and further therapy and support were spelled out. If I could, I tried to make sure that referrals were already done and the client had attended at least one appointment with the new service. I had the client sign the plan, agreeing to follow up on all recommendations. I gave them a copy and I kept a copy in their file. If they called back to come back to treatment, I would pull the discharge plan and see if they had followed it. If not, they were told to go back to the plan and put it in place and only then, if they couldn't manage, would we be willing to have them return to treatment. There had to be some accountability. This couldn't just be the go-to place when they decided they couldn't manage their lives. They had to have tried to live differently. They also had the option of second stage housing after treatment, so this should have been a successful plan.

The director of the treatment center where I was working as a volunteer decided at one point that she was leaving. She had very strong ethics regarding the way clients were treated. When she found out that one of the staff involved in the men's second stage houses was using clients to sell a product he was involved in, she gave the ultimatum that either this man be fired, or she would quit. She quit. I respected her decision, and I hoped that I would become a person who held my values as strongly as her. That she ended up quitting should have spelled out what I could expect from this world going forward. This was an ongoing problem in the staffing of these places. There was a lot of unethical behavior. By the time I left the field of addiction I would have seen absolutely every type of unethical behavior possible.

The other disturbing issue at this center was the unhealthiness of the staff. The house manager was clearly not healthy. He would call the clients drunks and be very derogatory toward them, meanwhile he was actively gambling. At one point he blocked the doorway of my small office and told me that all I needed was a good "fuck." He was eventually let go from his job after I had left.

I was hired by the treatment center just after the new director was hired. I had still been on long term disability from the bank, which had found in my favor in the investigation into the sexual assault. I had told them at one point to just stop paying me because I wasn't planning on going back to the bank, but I believed they insisted I continue getting support because of the findings in the case against my boss. I had a video recording and a taped conversation with my boss that would have made it very difficult for them not to find in my favor. When I was hired at the Men's Treatment Center, I resigned from the job officially. I received a letter from them stating they had found in my favor.

I worked for the treatment center for two and a half years while I had been completing a BA in Psychology. The cook at the center was taking a course at Algonquin College in addiction counseling, and he was seeing some of the clients individually. The government had become involved in a restructuring project aimed at overhauling the addiction treatment world. Everyone was nervous about this because it could mean reduced funding and loss of jobs and programs. This was around 1994. Up to this point, agencies who offered residential services were paid for everybody in a bed. Clients weren't assessed according to the best treatment for them because, at the time I don't think anyone really knew what the best treatment was. Everyone was vying for treatment dollars in order to survive. The government came in and decided which agency would provide what services, whether youth residential or outpatient, men's residential or outpatient, women's residential or outpatient or co-ed. They also determined how many employees each place could have. There was a plethora of evidence-based treatment models that were also put forward.

It's also important to put forward that the subject of compassion fatigue had also surfaced at this time. We were working with people who had experienced horrible childhoods and had been deeply traumatized by them. We were offered a group through one of the universities to allow us to process some of what we were being exposed to on a daily basis. Initially it was supposed to be the whole staff, but management chose to step back to give the employees a space to talk without their employer being present. We had already heard at this point that there would be cuts to staff. I began to realize that I would most likely be cut from the staff since I had been the last person hired. This hurt me because I had really put a lot into the center.

They had wanted to remodel the Relapse Prevention Program, and I had been working on this because no one seemed to have the time, and I really enjoyed doing this kind of work. As I attended the compassion fatigue group, I brought this forward. I knew that I was going to lose my job. At some point I was asked to train the guy who was the cook at the time to run the Relapse Prevention group, but still no one had announced who was going to get cut. I knew, of course, that I wasn't training this guy for nothing; I was training him to take my job. That is, in fact, what happened. What I did for the center was irrelevant. The fact that I had been delivering this program for over two years was irrelevant. I would train the person who would take my job, and I would leave.

I had left the second stage house just prior to this, and I

was living with two people who had lived at the house with me. I was also still seeing the adult child counselor, and I had been seeing a psychoanalyst that someone had recommended to me. I was over two years drug and alcohol-free when I left the house and was close to four years when I lost my job. I was still undergoing medication adjustments to balance my depression and agitation. I was still experiencing chronic suicidal ideation. I was still cutting myself. I was now unemployed, and after my unemployment ran out, I had to cash in on a Registered Retirement Savings Plan I had taken out when I terminated my bank job. It was a very stressful time for me. A job became available at the second stage house where I had been living previously and I worked there for a short time before they hired someone else. This was associated with the place I had been working at.

The addiction field is a rather incestuous field in that there are a lot of connections between the various agencies. The person they hired at the second stage house was the receptionist for the adult child counselor I was seeing. She was a woman who had a lot of years in recovery. She also had a significant trauma history. She had worked with my counselor as a receptionist for many years. She must have also been taking some sort of education to work in the field because she wanted to become a co-owner of the counseling service where she worked. This was not agreed to, and she had applied for the job at the second stage house.

The adult child counselor had also previously worked at the residential treatment program where I first did my treatment. She also seemed to know about things that were going on at the second stage house and the treatment center where I had been living and working. To make it all muddier, one of my roommates was the sponsee of the woman who had been working with my adult child counselor. In twelve-step groups you ask someone to be your sponsor in the program, and they do step work with you and support you in your recovery. They are the sponsor, and you are the sponsee.

Before I left the job there had also been something going on with the counselor from the second stage house who I had the transference with. There was something that had put her job at risk. I was warned by the new director that I was not to get involved in what was going on, which I assured her I was fine with because I had cut off contact with her by that point. This is what made the job become available. I was also receiving calls from people in the twelve-step program asking me to support her. If you find this at all confusing, you should try to be in the middle of it. I think my head would spin as I came to know more and more about the interconnections between all the players. I never really figured out what was going on in this situation.

The following is a diagram of the agencies I had contact with in my first two years of recovery:

Mental health hospital with a Residential Addiction Treatment Program

↓

Women's Second Stage Home (owned by the Men's Treatment Center)

↓

Men's Treatment Center (Relapse Prevention Program)

↓

Adult Child Counselor (Independent Counseling Service)

↓

Outpatient Women's Treatment Center

One other incident concerns the counselor that I had the transference with from the second stage house. She called me once to ask me to help her do an intervention with one of the women that I had known when I lived at the house. This woman was severely damaged and had lived a hard life. She had lost custody of her son when I first met her but was now living with her son and another guy. The counselor was concerned about her because she had relapsed, and she wanted her to go to treatment. She felt she could find somewhere to have the boy taken care of while she went for treatment so she would not lose her son.

This Counselor had a lot of issues around the notion of motherhood and what happens to women who are addicted and have children. She had negative experiences around her own young son when she had been using. She envisioned an underground group that would help addicted women keep their children while they went to treatment and that this would keep this out of the eye of child services. I made the mistake of saying I would accompany her.

When we got to the woman's place, we saw her son playing outside on his bike. We asked him to come to his place, and we went in to talk to the woman, who was noticeably drunk. There were bottles of pills on the table. We tried to convince her to go to treatment, but she refused.

We told her we would have to have the child removed from her care if she did not agree. The boy became very distraught at this point and began to cry, yelling at his mother that every time she drank, he had to leave and why couldn't she just not drink? It was absolutely heartbreaking.

She made him a plate of beans and wieners and I sat at the little table with him. My heart was breaking as well. Tears were falling down my face as I looked at this little guy who had no say in his life. The counselor called the police in order to get permission to take him out of this place because, with all the beer and pills, it was clearly an unsafe environment.

The police came, and she took the boy into her care. He took his hamster with him and placed the cage on his lap when he took a seat in her car. He was about seven years old.

I suggested that she stop at my place and bring him in. I had a big rabbit at the time, and I thought that he deserved something kind at that moment. The rabbit was very responsive to him, and I saw him smile for a moment. I remember giving him a long hug before they left.

The counselor called me afterwards. She had taken the boy to her house. She said she was going to take him back to his mother's the next day and try and get her to change her mind.

I thought she was crazy. We had just watched this little boy's heart break, and she wanted to go back over there and dangle him in front of her like bait. I couldn't accept that for a second. I called the Children's Aid Society and told them where we had picked the boy up from and where he was now. I gave them the counselor's address and told them what she was planning on doing. She was not taking the child into account, and I couldn't allow her to do that to him. I knew they would go to her place and take the child into custody.

I would find out much later that they had taken him into care that day. The counselor left me a nasty message, but later she called and apologized to me. I ran into the woman many years later, and she told me that she did go to treatment after her son was taken into care, and she did get him back. She thanked me for what I did that day and said her son had just recently mentioned me and talked about meeting my big rabbit. I was glad it had worked out for both of them.

What struck me about the counselor was it never landed on her for a minute how she was affecting the little boy. She was so focused on the mother role she forgot about the child and his feelings. This was clearly about her own issues.

It is clear that some of the dangers of working in this field and having your own history lie in the fact that you can hurt the people you are supposed to be helping. I continued to get professional help for the first seventeen years of my recovery. I did so because I knew I was not well. I had been terribly affected by my family life. I knew that I needed to work on these issues, or they would impact my work with my clients.

I remember running into this counselor years later, and she asked me how long I was planning to go to therapy. I told her that I would be going until I was well. I was not willing to settle for anything less.

I often wonder why I just didn't give up. I remained haunted by suicidal ideation for seventeen years into my recovery. It was only when they finally found the right medication combination that the thoughts finally subsided. I remember when they first went away, I was just waiting for them to come back. I couldn't believe that after all these years of having them as a constant unwanted hitchhiker in my life, they had finally fallen away. It was perhaps the most profound change that I experienced, not discounting all the therapy that had opened my eyes and all it had taught me about myself and humanity in general. Therapy was perhaps the greatest education that I have ever received.

Just prior to losing my job, I thought that it might be a good time to go and do some family work and I called and registered to take the family program at a hospital out of the city. It was a five-day residential program. While I was there, I had a knock on my room door at about 1:30 in the morning. When I answered the door, one of the other people taking the program with me insisted that I needed to come with her because there was something wrong with one of the others. I followed her to this woman's room, the lights were off, and someone was about to get into the bed with her. I told her to stop. It was clear by this woman's behavior that she was in some sort of flashback and unaware of where she was.

A male attendant came to the door, and I told him that having a male go to her would not be advisable and that they needed to get a woman. I went over to her bed and sat on the side and began telling her where she was. She stated that she was in a closet and her uncle was coming, and she was in great distress. I just kept a calm voice and kept telling her my name and where she was. I finally asked her if she could sit up in her bed and she was able to do this. It was clear she was coming out of it. When I knew she was awake enough, I asked her if we could turn on the lights in her room, and she agreed. I then suggested that we get up and have a cup of tea. It all took about forty-five minutes, and at that time no employee of the hospital came back.

I wondered to myself how I ended up in this situation but then I had, and would often, find myself in this situation. I would like to make it clear that I am not mentioning this to say that I thought I had this great amount of knowledge. I just think that there are a lot of situations where you have to ask yourself, what the hell are the professionals doing, or where the hell are the professionals?

This woman was having a trauma flashback of sexual abuse by a male relative and needed someone to help her come out of it. Why were there no female staff on that night that could have come to help her out. No one ever came back to offer any help. We all eventually went back to bed. I can't remember anything much being said the next day.

My Second Job in the Addiction Field

I had received a referral from the Family Program to see a doctor who worked in my city. I called him up. He was nice and appeared to be knowledgeable about addiction and how it affected the family. He made another appointment with me, and I went, but forty-five minutes past the time for my appointment, I left because I had to go back to work. I didn't bother booking another appointment because if he was that late seeing his clients it wouldn't work for me.

Oddly enough, he contacted me and asked if I would be interested in joining a group of people who were interested in designing an addiction program for women and their babies. I found this interesting because it made a lot of sense. I worked on this project with him and others for about four months when he offered me a job.

He was planning on turning his office into a counseling center for people with addictions, and he wanted to know if I wanted to work there. I agreed. Once more I ask myself, why did a doctor who I was originally sent to for counseling hire me to work as a counselor? I would eventually find out that he was in recovery from addiction as well.

I would work with him for over four years. Originally, I really admired him. He was smart and caring. I was very interested in neuroscience and the brain and so was he. We would have many interesting conversations over the four and a half years I worked with him before the whole thing took a turn down a rather dark alley.

When he set up his center, I think he envisioned it to be a

fee-for-service arrangement, but people who have devastated their lives with addiction often don't work and can't pay for services. When this became the problem, he decided that he could bill the (OHIP) Ontario Health Insurance Plan for the sessions we had with the clients. As long as he did a check-in with them this would pay us $20.00 an hour for our clients. I have never been sure whether this was something that OHIP would have sanctioned, and it came up much later as an issue.

I ran a couple of groups, and I saw about twenty-five clients a week. I enjoyed the work, and I kept upgrading my education as I had been doing all along, by taking many workshops and attending conferences to improve my skills. I loved learning, so I always looked for education in new therapies and treatments that would make me a better counselor. I was still seeing the psychoanalyst at the time.

A note on psychoanalysis: I attended sessions with my psychoanalyst four times a week for eleven years. I believe, in my early recovery, it was helpful because I had a lot of contact with him, and I needed it. He was a psychiatrist, so he was OHIP-covered. Each session cost between $100.00 and about $110.00. I once added up the total cost of the eleven years and wondered, if OHIP realized what the cost of trying to correct a broken childhood was, would they be more interested in prevention? This therapy did not make me much better. He rarely said much, as is the way of analysis, and lying on a couch, trying to meander through some attempt to say whatever came to my mind, eventually became nothing but a source of endless frustration for me.

I stayed because I was desperate for some connection and some way to try and get better. When we ended the therapy, he told me that, despite the fact that I had never fully engaged in the analysis, I had managed to drag myself some distance. Not exactly a glowing report. I've always wanted to call him up and tell him that I got a lot better after I stopped going to him, but that would be a rather petty thing to do. He was a lifeline for many years.

I'd also like to mention the doctor I was seeing for my psychiatric medications. I had seen several psychiatrists regarding meds, and I spent some time with one in particular. He worked out of one of the hospitals and he also had a private practice. I would see him for the most part at the hospital. In the last year that I was working for the doctor, I had been having increasing problems with my depression and suicidal ideation. I had long periods where I would be in a mixed manic state, and I could not sleep. Being suicidal at these times was excruciating.

Working most often distracted me and that was helpful. At one point my meds psychiatrist decided to take me off all my meds to make a change in them. This caused the mania to increase to a point where I was unable to sleep, and the agitation that resulted in the night became unbearable. I was constantly thinking of killing myself, and there were times at work when I canceled all my clients but stayed in my office with the door locked because I was afraid to go home in case, I killed myself. It had clearly gotten out of hand.

I called up my doctor and his receptionist answered. I explained that I was really having problems with suicidal thoughts, and I couldn't wait another two weeks to see my doctor before my appointment came up. She said she would call me back. When she called back, she said he didn't have any appointment times and not only that, but he would have to push my appointment back another two weeks. I made it clear to her that I could not wait that long and that I needed to see him as I was on no medications, and I was clearly in distress. She asked me if I saw anyone for counseling. I said I saw a psychoanalyst, but he did not prescribe medications. She asked if he was a psychiatrist, and I said yes but repeated that he did not prescribe medications. She said that since I was already seeing a psychiatrist, I could not see my doctor at all and hung up the phone. I'm hoping again that you might be asking yourself what the hell.

I can't begin to tell you how distressing this was for me. I now had no doctor to deal with my medications, and I was in a state of mixed mania and depression and was highly suicidal. She didn't even suggest that I might want to go to emergency. I saw this as the end. I couldn't go on with the way I felt. I wrote a letter to that doctor saying that I could not manage the way I was, and now that he had refused to see me, I could not go on. I took a bottle of trazadone pills which were antidepressants often prescribed for sleeping issues and about ten clonazepam that my medical doctor had prescribed for me because I was struggling with agitation.

After I took the pills, I kept trying to come up with an alternate plan. I called my medical doctor, and the receptionist said she was busy and could she call me back. I said it would be too late, and she clearly got the message because my doctor appeared on the phone. I told her what I had done, and, by this point, I was feeling the effects of the sedation. She sent an ambulance to my home, and I was taken to the hospital. I spent the day at the hospital after ingesting charcoal to induce vomiting. I left at about ten to go home. I never saw anyone there to address my psychological state. The next day continued like any other day.

The psychiatrist's office that had refused to see me eventually called me up at some point and asked me to come in for an appointment, and I went. He had received the readout from a heart test they had done on me when I was taken to the hospital. He asked me what it was. I said that I had tried to kill myself. He told me that if I did that again he would not see me. I figured that was a good possibility.

He also received the letter I wrote to him after taking the pills. Had I been psychologically better I would have made a complaint against him, but I was at the mercy of the people who might have the power to help me, and I knew that I couldn't do it myself. He would not be the person who helped me find the right medication, but thankfully I would live long enough to find that person.

Again, I point out the complete irresponsibility of this doctor and his receptionist, who was his wife. I had made it very clear how urgent my situation was and why I needed to see the doctor. The doctor had taken me off all my medication, and I had a diagnosis of bipolar disorder with severe depression. I was suffering from mixed mania at the time; I could not sleep, and I had constant suicidal ideation. This receptionist did not even relay the message to the doctor or suggest that I go to the hospital. If I hadn't had the wherewithal to call my medical doctor, who had been my doctor for years, I might well be dead.

I am very grateful to my medical doctor, who has always been a wonderful and diligent doctor. She has retired and I was sad when she did because I owed her so much for her kindness and her great care over the many years of my life. Her name was Dr. Karen McIntosh.

Back to the doctor's office where I was working. There were things along the way that began suggesting that all was not well with the doctor. He had a lot of clients because he was really good at getting people put on disability for their addiction. He always had problems with timeliness. He could be quite late seeing his patients and I was to discover why. He had a receptionist who booked clients for him and then he was also making appointments with patients himself. It wasn't that he didn't know he had clients being booked for him; it was that if someone contacted him and wanted to see him, he'd agree. This was a constant source of aggravation for his patients, but if they were relying on him to fill out paperwork for disability, they'd put up with it.

At some point he decided to move offices, and he had his patients help him separate rooms into offices, put up walls and paint them. This was an ethical violation. You don't have the right to have your clients or patients do work for you for free. Things at the new office began to deteriorate rather quickly.

If he was late before, it now became ridiculous. Not only did he double book but he had to touch base with our clients as well, for us to be paid. The atmosphere in the waiting room began to shift noticeably. It became much more aggressive. At one point I had to go out of my office and confront a patient who was swearing and threatening the receptionist. I had a client with a serious trauma history who was being triggered by this man's performance. I managed to get him to sit down, but no one else had come out to intervene.

What finally came to light was that he had decided to start his own idea of harm reduction, and he was prescribing morphine to people with an opiate addiction. He needed to get a special certificate to prescribe methadone, so he decided to prescribe morphine. I also noticed that many people who had not been opiate addicts were now being prescribed morphine.

The morphine began to show up on the streets, and the patients in the waiting room became very different from what they used to be. This was the beginning of the end, but it would take a long time, and the situation would have to get really bad before anything would be done to shut all this down.

One thing I began to notice was the people in charge of getting people healthy were not very healthy. I reached a point where I knew I had to do something, and I knew that I needed to leave this place. So many things had happened that I could not just stand there and watch as it continued. I was burnt out myself.

The attempt to recover from my own mental health issues had yet to succeed, and the stress in the office was aggravating it more. I applied for disability on the basis of my mental health. It had been determined that I had bipolar disorder type two. While I was waiting for the verdict on my application, I began to write a letter to the College of Physicians documenting the things that I had seen going on in the office. It ended up being an eleven-page letter.

The following are some of what I saw going on in his office:

The doctor had two examination rooms to see patients. He would see one while another person waited in the next office. He would leave his prescription pad out where it was visible, so many went missing. He would take people's discarded meds and keep them in a cupboard in case someone needed meds but couldn't afford them. More than once, I found clients shopping in this cupboard before I told them to get out of it.

He had stopped recording information in the client's files, and the files lay in piles all around his offices. He was prescribing all sorts of psychiatric medications to his clients, which caused some serious problems at times. Since he wasn't documenting what he was doing, clients could end up on as much as thirty medications at a time. Pharmacies had begun to call because they couldn't understand why he had people on various combinations. They also became concerned when all the morphine prescriptions kept appearing. There were some individuals admitted to hospital because of the many medications he had them on. Despite this no one made a formal complaint.

There was also a point where it became obvious that he was taking drugs. He had gone to treatment previously when he had become addicted as a doctor. It was his behavior that made me believe that he had to be taking something. Mind you, he worked ridiculously long hours, so he could have been exhausted from overworking, but it looked more like drugs. He would show up in one of my groups to do a quick check-in, and he would ask one patient how she was doing and, a moment later, he would ask her again, as if he had forgotten that he had already checked in with her. One time he came in and he was wearing a loafer on one foot and a running shoe on the other. It would have been funny if it weren't for all the people who were negatively affected and for those who died.

There are two people that I knew who died. One young man died of a morphine overdose on the street. I knew him from the twelve-step rooms. He misdiagnosed another woman, and when she finally saw someone else, she had cancer, and it had progressed to the stage where it would be fatal. He would never be held responsible for these two deaths, but I would come to see other examples where a doctor's actions directly brought about a person's death, and it seemed not to really matter. It seems that there are many different loopholes you can find to alleviate responsibility simply by being a doctor.

There was a young man with severe depression and a trauma history that I was seeing. He needed serious medical intervention for his depression, and I went to the doctor, explaining that he needed a referral. The doctor prescribed him an antidepressant. The antidepressant was not working, and I went to the doctor again regarding this. He changed the prescription. This young man hanged himself in a very public place after leaving me a suicide note that I did not receive until after his death. It was devastating to me. I had to call the police because I could not get an answer at his home. They called back and told me he had already died. I finished my workday and went home. Later in the week I was mentioning that the death had really shaken me up, and he asked, "Are you not over that yet?" Once again, I'm hoping you are very disturbed about this because I certainly was. This young man was about thirty years old, and he was very bright, and he should not have died. His death had a profound impact on me. I have never forgotten him and it is unlikely that I ever will.

This hastened my leaving this office, but there were other things that were hard not to be appalled by. He once told a neighbor of one of our clients that she wasn't as fucked up as her. One of the counselors at the center had taken one of my clients to his home after offering to drive her home. Once there he offered to show her pornographic films from his collection. She was a person who had experienced sexual abuse, and he just happened to be working with her abuser. I wrote a letter to the doctor explaining what had happened and asking him to take action. The doctor told the counselor that he could not see clients at the office, but he could see them at his home. He also continued to refer female clients to him. This was just unacceptable.

One of the other counselors received a call from a woman disturbed by her husband, who had locked himself up in a bedroom and who had a gun. She transferred the call to the doctor, who told the woman that he didn't have the time to deal with the situation. He was well aware of this man because he had him in one of his groups, and other members had expressed concerns about being in the group with this man because of his aggression. The counselor came to me upset and asked what she should do. I told her to call 911 because, obviously, the situation called for that level of response. When he was apprehended, they found a large number of prescribed medications from the doctor in the trunk of his car. Despite this, the doctor wasn't investigated.

The doctor also began to collect a lot of plants in his office, and I mean more plants than seemed to make any sense. There were plants everywhere. He looked like he'd become a florist. The number of plants made his offices look like there was something wrong with him.

A friend of mine who was seeing the doctor as a counselor came to my office one day, and she had just had a cyst removed from her leg by the doctor. It was bleeding through the bandage. Apparently, he had cut it out before he realized that he did not have any sutures. He had bandaged it up, but it was clear that it needed stitches. I told her to go back and show him it was bleeding through the bandage. He re-bandaged it, but this was just not going to work. She went back again, and he told her he didn't have time for it. I told her she had to go to a clinic and get stitches. I was afraid she'd go home and bleed to death. She agreed to go to a clinic and had four stitches put in. They didn't want to touch it, as it was another doctor's work, but it was clear the bleeding wouldn't stop. I'm hoping someone is also wondering why any of these medical people along the way hadn't thought to make a complaint.

He also gave an ointment to one of the other counselors who had an eye infection. When it worsened, she went to an eye doctor who informed her that not only was the medication six months out of date, but it was an entirely wrong medication and could have caused blindness if she continued to use it. She never thought of making a complaint.

I was working with a couple who had some serious addiction issues and a young child about eighteen months old. I was working in conjunction with the Children's Aid Society because the infant had been taken into care. The male partner showed up one day. He was in obvious pain and said this was from a gunshot wound he received from people who were after him. He also had long red scratches down one side of his face because his partner had gotten into a fight with him. I wrote two very detailed letters explaining why I did not think that the child should be returned to the couple at this time. I gave copies of the letter to the doctor. He also saw the male partner the day I saw him. I got a telephone call from the CAS asking what had happened because the doctor had written a glowing letter stating the couple was doing well in recovery and should have their son returned to them. I went to see the doctor and asked how, after reading my two letters, he had written a letter to support them to get their child back.

He said he hadn't read my letters and stated, "I guess I made a mistake." I have to ask again how someone can be in this man's position and be able to get away with this? There was no way to undo what he had done because he was the doctor.

There was a woman that I had worked with who had three young children. I ran into her years later when her children were adults and resumed therapy with her. She described how she had continued to see this doctor and that he had her taking a large number of medications, so many that she found herself constantly sleeping rather than being able to care for her young children. When she repeatedly told him that she was having difficulty being able to stay awake, he would tell her she needed to keep taking the medications or she could end up killing herself, as her brother had, and then her children would have no mother. Her children still recall her being in this drugged state, barely able to be there for them. She said she took the medications because he was the doctor, and she thought he knew what he was doing. Looking back, she realizes that he didn't because these medications did not help her. They robbed her of many years of her children's lives.

I saw this over and over when he had clients on so many medications that they could not function at all; he had stopped keeping his records up to date, and he often did not even remember what he had his clients on. What is maddening is that people like him could get away with doing things like this, which had such serious effects on the lives of others, and they would never be held accountable for the damage they caused. I saw this over and over throughout the work I did.

At the height of the morphine project, we had people shooting up in the building's public washrooms outside of the office, and things began to get very rough inside the office. The attempts to steal went up. Threats in the waiting room went up. The clients were more aggressive. The wait times were longer. The doctor looked more and more like there was something wrong with him. He was working from 8:00 am to 11:00 pm. He was working weekends. His wife was in the office more often. He was failing to bill OHIP. Some staff had jumped ship. It looked like things were going downhill. Many clients were way too overprescribed.

I started telling him he should go for treatment. He didn't like that very much, but I could see there was something very wrong with him. He needed some help. That's what made me write the letter, and that's part of what I said in the letter. I had begun to think he was using morphine. It's the only thing that could make sense of his chaotic behavior. I don't know for sure what it was because I left by the time I sent the letter in.

The College kindly sent him a copy of the letter I wrote them. They never told me that. I found out from someone that was still there. They never considered that doing that could have put me in any danger. They never let me know that they had sent my letter to him. Had I still been at the office, I would have been in danger.

I documented eleven pages of serious behaviors that involved this doctor in the letter I sent to the College of Physicians. They even sent people to photograph the office because, believe me, it merited being photographed. This was in 1999–2000.

He would not have to surrender his medical license until seventeen years later, and only after continuous violations of the college's restrictions on him. I have to ask why he was able to cause the damage that he did and it would take so long for this kind of action to be taken against him.

I'd like to say the College of Psychologists was more than happy threatening to take Jordon Peterson's license away for things he said on social media, but this man could cause deaths, threaten lives and flood the streets with pharmaceutical morphine and barely get a slap on the wrist. I'm rather confused about where our moral leaning lies.

It was common in the addiction field for things to go very, very wrong and for nothing to happen in response. Since many people with lived experience worked in the field, it wasn't uncommon for some of them to relapse. I always wondered why there wasn't any testing demanded for employees who were in recovery because, in my mind, that would have been reasonable.

The other common occurrence was the tendency for sexual impropriety with clients. That one seemed to show up everywhere. I don't know how many times I heard about people who had slept with their clients. I would have thought that one would be an obvious thing not to do, but surprisingly it seemed to not stop anyone from doing it.

Taking a Break from Working in the Field

I had been living with a woman that I had moved in with after leaving the second stage house. There had initially been three of us, but the other woman left after we all had a falling out. I was still suffering from the attachment issue I had from my unhealthy relationship with my mother. When unhealthy is the only relationship you know, you keep repeating it until you find a way to heal it.

I repeated this with my roommate. I attached to her in a way that felt like survival. I treated her like my mother had treated me. I needed her to be there all the time for me. I was still so wounded, and even though I knew what was happening, I didn't know how to stop it. We lived together for seven years until she found a relationship with a man she was working with. I was not the person she needed in her life, and I caused a lot of emotional harm to her before it all blew up and she moved out.

What I really needed was to live alone until I could live alone with myself and manage. I have never lived with someone since then. It took a long time before the pain of my aloneness subsided. I have never tried to get into a relationship with a man again either. I came to realize that I just did not know how to be in a relationship, romantic or otherwise.

I have felt alone at times because I feel like I am a ship without a place to dock. I have accepted it for the most part, but there are still times when I feel very much alone.

I lost my sister to cancer when I was fifty and she was fifty-one. At that moment I felt like I had lost contact with a person who loved me unconditionally. She and I had become good friends in our adulthood, and she had been there for me on more than one occasion. I could always call her, and she was there for me. I loved her deeply, and I miss her terribly. When I feel the greatest pain in my life, I feel I am alone. I have few close friends in my life today. Those that I do are often busy with their own lives and family.

The silence in which I live my personal life is sometimes so loud it hurts. I manage it by engaging in a myriad of creative activities. I draw and paint, take photos and write poetry constantly. In this way I am trying to engage in a conversation where there is no one to converse with. Most often I feel like an artist without an audience. I think part of me wants to leave something behind that says I was here. I've self-published fifteen books on art, photography, and poetry. My creativity is the only child I could give birth to and the only part of me I will leave behind. I work hard to come to peace with this.

I took just over a year off working in the addiction field, part of which I worked in a job that had nothing to do with anything I had ever done before. It paid minimum wage, and I worked from 11:00 pm until 7:00 am constructing fiber optic switches. My mind needed a break, but even here addiction would make an appearance. One of the guys who worked the shift I did would get progressively more drunk and crude as the night wore on. I found it very difficult to work near this guy, listening to the sexually offensive things he said all night. I finally asked the very young man who was managing our section to do something and so he moved him away from where I was working. His alcohol use was never addressed. I was laid off when the company went out of business.

I applied for a position teaching at a private college. I started with one course and this turned into a whole program in Addiction and Community Service Work. It was a trial by fire, and you either learned how to teach or you wouldn't last long.

I worked there for nine years. If anything, it really solidified my knowledge of addiction, psychology, counseling, and pharmacology. I had to be able to teach and explain everything I was teaching. Initially, it was a lot of work because I had to learn all the material I was going to teach with enough clarity that I could answer any questions and elaborate on the material from real-life situations.

It was a rough start as I tried to navigate the world of a private college. The aim of these places is obviously to make money, so there was always a big push to sign people up for their courses, and the salespeople were under pressure to do this. It was like if you had a pulse you could sign up for whatever program. That posed some serious problems in the classroom where the ability of the students ranged from competent to clearly incapable.

The other issue with this kind of program is it touches on some pretty sensitive areas, so if the person is not emotionally stable, you could have some serious issues surfacing. The size of the classes ranged from about twelve to thirty students. There were sixteen subjects, and they were taught one at a time for five hours a day with two breaks. I taught from 8:00 am to 1:00 pm.

At first, I was almost eaten alive by the students. I needed to learn how to control a classroom of people who didn't have the best classroom habits. I eventually learned classroom management, but that didn't mean there weren't regular problems that popped up when one or more of the students were unwell enough to derail the room.

I have always believed that if you are going to do a job, then you should do your best. This course was supposed to prepare people to get an entry level position in an addiction or social-related agency. In my mind, that meant that they needed to be educated and suitable enough to do the work. It was a question of ethics, and I'd seen enough ethical violations up to that point to last me a lifetime. It would be unethical to put people through a course where they were clearly not capable and pass them.

The school wanted us to get people through the course to completion with no dropouts or failures. Ontario Student Assistance Program (OSAP) which provided loans to students demanded that the students be in the class every day, so attendance became crucial. If the students had been screened for the course, it probably wouldn't have been impossible, but several of the students were often ill-suited and had no study skills or basic English writing skills.

Many had serious interpersonal issues and, at times, I would have to break up arguments that escalated into students cursing at each other. Once, the director came to my office to inform me that two of my students were physically fighting in the mall as if I was supposed to go out and break it up. I suggested that she call security.

I taught a course on the family, and addiction and dysfunction in the family, and every time I got to that course there would be a fallout. I had students lashing out at me when asked to do a genogram of their family because it just brought up so many undealt with issues. I explained to them over and over that if they had not done any work on themselves, then they would be at constant risk of being triggered and harming the person with whom they were working. They could not go into this type of work with a lot of unhealed wounds of which they weren't even aware.

I stressed the importance of them getting counseling for themselves. I used my own examples to show them how you can be triggered by something that you were unaware of before that moment. I told them I was still in therapy and had been throughout the time I was working in the field. I talked about transference and countertransference. Despite my best efforts, the nature of the people being accepted into the course posed a constant problem. I tried to explain to the college over and over that they could not just put any person into a course like this. I spoke to the salespeople, but no one listened, and this was a constant issue throughout the nine years that I was there.

Another aspect of my job was that, at the end of the course, I was supposed to set up a placement for the students. This was another serious issue for me. If I recommended a student for a placement and they went there and were a disaster, that would reflect back on me. Again, the ethical aspect of this did not sit right with me.

I would not recommend every student I worked with for a job if they were not suitable for this kind of work. If they harmed someone at their placement, I would feel like I had put the client at risk by placing an unsuitable person there.

In fact, there was a situation that clinched it for me. One of my female students was in a placement with young male offenders. She was dismissed from her placement for engaging in questionable behavior with one of the clients. That was the deciding moment for me. I made it clear that I would not be arranging placements with anyone I felt was not suitable to be in a placement.

The school tried to insist that this was part of my job, and I made it clear that I also owed the community agencies the ethical position of not sending them any students who could end up harming their clients. At some point there was a second Addiction and Community Worker Course offered in the afternoon, but when it came down to placements many agencies would only take the students that I recommended because they knew that I would have made sure that they were suitable.

I once had two drug dealing gang members who showed

up to take the course. It was clear that they looked like the part. I was struck by what in hell the salespeople were doing when they signed these two guys up. I taught on the first day, just really giving the students an idea of the courses we would be covering and talking about addiction and its effect on people and society.

One of these guys came up at the end of the day and told me that he didn't think too much of me when he walked in, but now, having heard me, he thought I was someone he could talk to. I wasn't sure what to make of that.

At some point, a little later on, at the beginning of the course, he asked me if he could talk to me. He told me that he gave some cocaine to his best friend one night, and he went home, used it and then killed himself. He became very emotional as he spoke about this. His friend had been someone he really cared about, and he couldn't get over thinking that if he hadn't given him the cocaine, maybe he wouldn't have killed himself. We talked for a while, and then he said that he wouldn't see me again unless he found a way to change his life.

He left with the guy that started the class with him and never came back. I believe he had come to the course to try and deal with this tragedy. It seems like an extreme thing to do, to sign up for a one-year course to talk to someone, but as strange as that sounds, I don't think it is uncommon.

I believe that a lot of people signed up for the course because they themselves were struggling, and they thought if they took the course maybe they could figure out what was wrong and then fix it.

They may not have realized it at the time, but I do believe that this was often what was sitting underneath. I think it's a sad commentary on society where those who have been injured by the circumstances of their lives have to sign up for a course in order to find some measure of self-understanding.

At times I felt like I was doing group counseling with sometimes up to twenty-seven people at a time. I could say the same about myself when I took psychology. I was trying to understand myself, my family and the people in my life.

There were people who were competent in the class. They often lost patience with all of the nonsense that could occur in the classroom, and there was a constant need to remind students that they were there to learn. I'm sure many teachers can tell you the same stories about people on their phones, playing games on their computers, or constantly talking while you're trying to teach. I got better and better at managing these situations as I went along. The unhealthy students were often the most difficult because many of them should not have been accepted into the course, but they had taken a loan out to pay for it, so they had a right to be in the classroom.

I spent a lot of time teaching study skills and creating study guides for each exam. I was forced to offer rewrite after rewrite because they couldn't be allowed to fail. On written assignments, plagiarism was the rule, not the exception. I don't know how many times I entered the first line of their assignment into the search engine only to have the whole thing appear on the internet. I would print out the internet article and hand it back to them with a zero, telling them to do it again.

In a resume writing class, many of them wrote their cover letter in texting language and did not understand what the issue was. I taught grammar which was painful because most of them did not know anything about grammar. It was a very difficult situation because most of them genuinely wanted to do well.

I sat in on a colleague's class once because he had to be away, and the class was writing an exam. He told me that there was one student who made people nervous because he had some really dark things written on the cover of his notebook. Suddenly, in the middle of the exam he stood up and made a very loud guttural sound and headed for the door. I followed him out of concern, and he had stepped through the exit to outside and was returning. I asked him if he was OK, and he said he was having feelings.

He came back to the classroom, and I asked him to stay after the class ended so I could talk to him. As we talked after class it became obvious that he was suffering from some kind of psychosis. He talked to me for a while and then asked me if I could tell his parents what was happening to him. I called his parents and asked them to come and pick up their son and that they needed to take him to the emergency room at the hospital because he was clearly suffering from a mental health issue. He was admitted to the hospital with a psychotic depression, and his parents were very grateful that I had intervened.

My question is, he was clearly showing symptoms for some time while in my colleague's class. Why in hell did he not check into it further? How long was he just going to leave this young man suffering in his class without at least talking to him about what was going on with him? The young man was very open to talking and it hadn't been hard to talk to him. He eagerly asked me to help him. All he needed was someone to ask him what was happening and how he was feeling. My colleague worked as a counselor so he should have had the skills to do this.

I was teaching a soft skills class one day, which is a course that all students must take, so it included students who would go on to other courses. One of the salespersons dropped a woman off at the course. I recognized immediately that she was an active crack user. I ran out after the salesperson and caught up with her in the hallway. I asked her if she was unaware that this woman was high on crack. She said it's alright because she's not taking your course. I said once she gets the OSAP money she won't be taking anyone's course. I was often struck by the absolute foolishness of these salespeople. This was a perfect scam for an addicted person because all they had to do was hang around until they got the loan money, and then they would make a big score. They would not stay after that. They would use the money for drugs.

I won teacher of the year while working there and got a trip to the States because the college was an extension of an American college. I also had the opportunity to change the course and update material while I was there. We were eventually able to be recognized by the Addiction Certification Board for providing all the required education for certification. I learned a lot myself while there. It deepened my education, and nine years of repetition made me very knowledgeable in the field of addiction. Teaching counseling skills through experiential learning also deepened my counseling skills. Learning how to manage a classroom would come in handy later.

I was always involved in my own education with endless courses, workshops, and conferences. I took four years of experiential training in Gestalt therapy that was at the Post Graduate Level despite only having a BA. I would eventually spend many years studying psychodrama, first as a client and then as a trainee. I was very interested in trauma and spent years studying therapies for treating PTSD. I had an unquenchable thirst for knowledge. If I encountered something I didn't understand then I tried to find information on it. I loved searching for new concepts and conditions I had never encountered before. I always felt that if I was working with someone and I didn't know about what they were struggling with, then it was my duty to find out. I believed that was my ethical duty.

Once, when I was working at the doctor's office, I had a woman in one of my groups who was very difficult to have in the group. I can only describe my reaction as feeling annoyed with her all the time. The other group members were also losing patience with her. I thought to myself, why would someone keep doing things that obviously annoy people? I kept thinking that there must be something wrong with her.

No attempt at intervention worked. I thought maybe it was a learning thing, and if she went to some rehab for social behaviors, she could learn how to change this. I documented all of the behaviors that I was seeing in the group with her and sent off a referral to a rehab hospital. It would be pertinent to tell you that this woman was sixty years old and had a university degree. I say this because no one had ever addressed this issue for her. It's not like it just developed. She had this problem all of her life.

A while later she came in for an individual appointment, all excited. She announced, "I have Asperger's," with a big smile. She said, "All this time I thought it was just me, but I actually have a disorder." This woman had suffered social isolation all of her life. Why had no one up to this point ever asked themselves what was wrong? What could knowing that diagnosis have done for her in the way of self-understanding and access to services?

I had never heard of Asperger's, but I took the time to learn about it and then this woman made perfect sense to me. I have seen situation after situation like this. Why is one person's life not important enough to go the extra mile? Too often I have seen lives thrown away like they are of no significance. I have seen people die because professionals are unwilling to do their jobs, and the level of profession doesn't matter. It often seems like the higher you go up professionally, the more of these transgressions you find.

I had still been trying to find a solution to my suicidal ideation that had continued to plague me. I was also aware that I didn't relate well to my own gender. I had grown up having been treated like a male. I didn't understand women. I had never been a person that dressed in an overly feminine way. I never wore make-up or dresses. I didn't even understand how to be a woman. I genuinely didn't understand it. I sought some help with this and was referred to a psychiatrist who dealt with sexual disorders. I was referred for gender identity disorder. The first thing he asked me was if I wanted him to make me into a male. I was clear that wasn't the issue.

I ended up working with a counselor associated with him who really was helpful to me. The best thing that came out of the referral to him was he found the right medication combination to treat my suicidal ideation and mood disorder. It took some time and, at one point, he had put me on lithium, and I just could not function. I literally couldn't think. I waited to see him before stopping the lithium because I had this rule with myself that I would not make decisions about my meds without my doctor's input.

I've seen so many people have difficulties with their medications because they chose to stop them or change how much they were taking, and this almost always leads to bad results. I would have the same thoughts as everyone else about stopping my meds, but I chose to view those thoughts as a symptom and not to act on them. I also monitored myself daily when I was on new medications. I would keep a log of how I felt each day. It is one of the best ways for the doctor to gauge how your meds are working. They aren't with you every day, and if you don't keep track then you don't remember if there are changes over time. You can only tell them how you feel today.

When the suicide ideation left me, I was shocked. It was like someone had turned off a station in my mind that had been playing forever. I kept expecting it to return, and it just never did. It was a freedom that I was so appreciative of. The other thing about the meds that I was put on is that they did not blunt my emotions or numb me. I was left with all of my feelings and my energy. It's like it just turned things down from way too high to normal. I feel very grateful because not all people get this result.

I have been described as intense, and I would have to agree with that, but I believe that has always been part of me. I am still at risk when stress is too high, and I have to be aware of that. Being in the type of work that I do, that is often hard. Keeping healthy is a full-time job, and it involves finding enough activities that keep me in a safe place. When your life is constantly stressful you have to find things that allow you to release some of that. I am an artist, a poet, a writer, a researcher, and a photographer. These outlets provide me with ways to direct my frustration into something that creates and doesn't destroy. Again, I am lucky that I have been gifted with so many outlets and the creativity to engage in them all.

The other therapy that became important to me was Psychodrama. I had been curious about it since my first residential treatment, where I had not been able to take part due to my having been too overwhelmed by the film on the addicted family. I think I realized at that time even that this was a powerful way of really connecting to one's issues. I sought out the woman who had been doing this at that treatment center and she had by now left and was working out of a doctor's office. I wanted to learn how to do it professionally. She suggested that I try it as a client a few times before I decided to take any training. I would give this therapy credit for really resolving the lion's share of my trauma work. I participated in five psychodrama weekends as a client. It was very hard work, but it achieved amazing results. I have been in training with this woman since then. I always have reservations because I have always been a more introverted person, especially physically. I pushed myself because I wanted to grow in this area. I learned over time that it is healthy to do things that take you out of your comfort zone.

What happened working in the addiction field affected me very negatively. At the end of it all I was left with a deep depression that I still struggle with. It was a mistake to stay as long as I did, and what I experienced in those places impacted me heavily. People often tell me I must be proud of all the good that I did, but there was so much wrong with the places I worked that I was deeply impacted. Some of it was directly related to the way I was treated. I experienced very abusive workplaces. It wore me down and impacted my sense of self. It is hard to believe that people who worked in agencies that were supposed to help people could be so unkind to the people who worked for them. In many ways it replicated my abusive past. At one point, I tried going to the Human Rights Tribunal, but I had no one to support me through the process. I settled, but I could have gone much further, given all that had been done to me.

Back Into the Addiction Field

I returned to the addiction counseling field. For a time, I worked with high school kids and youth. A lot of the kids I saw came from troubled homes where addiction was common. I noticed that if the parents used drugs, then so did their kids. The thing with addiction is if you are using you don't want to be seen as doing something wrong, so you try to normalize it. One way to do that is to let your kids use as well. It sends the message that using is OK. Most of the parents used alcohol, but there was a growing number using pot. The message that everyone was sending is that pot is a safe drug, and if you're an adult certainly it is less damaging than other drugs.

If you are an adolescent, pot is not a safe drug. What I watched happen is how quickly pot use derailed a kid's chances of being successful in school. It affects memory and focus so anyone who is already struggling academically will often really be affected in school. The other threat was early onset psychosis. I worked with a number of kids who developed psychosis, and their continued pot use increased their mental breaks and often caused additional issues for them.

One young man I worked with became very derailed mentally from using pot. He quickly became a young man in crisis. His behavior became unpredictable and strange. Adolescence is a difficult time all by itself, but when you add in mental health issues brought on by drug use, things can become overwhelmingly difficult. This is more problematic because we are talking about young people who haven't got all the tools that they need to navigate the world yet. Adolescence is also made difficult by the tendency for them to be hard on each other. Teasing, bullying, rejection, and isolation can be difficult enough. This young man had experienced a great deal of rejection. When he became derailed, he experienced a lot of anger.

Eventually his odd behavior got him kicked out of school. This was followed by an arrest over a misunderstanding at an OC Transpo station where he had been a witness to a fight. The police wanted him to give them his bus pass because that was his only ID. He, in his unstable state, thought they were going to take it from him, so he resisted giving it to them. Everything quickly spiraled out of control, and he was arrested.

In court, the legal aid lawyer would not agree that he should be in a mental health court. I could not understand how she couldn't see how unstable he was. I asked if I could go down to see him when she went down to talk to him before court. I got to see how she determined that he could give her direction. She wrote innocent and guilty on a piece of paper. She pointed to each one, saying, 'Which do you want to plead?' He would be going off in all directions and would not be making much sense, and she would just continue to point at the two possible answers over and over until he finally chose one: innocent. This was her confirmation that he could participate in the legal process.

This was an example of the legal system unwilling to do its job. I had told this lawyer that my client was unwell. He had a form of autism, and he had used some spice, and this had affected his mental health considerably. He would often ramble about all sorts of things, but it wasn't clear that he understood what he was speaking about. He had Semantic Pragmatic Disorder, which meant he could absorb a great deal of information, but he would not necessarily understand it, so, although he could sound like he was very knowledgeable, he might have no idea about what he was talking about. He had been doing just that when she had asked him how he had wanted to plead. The only way she got an answer was by writing it on paper and constantly pointing to either one, then asking him which one until he finally gave her an answer she wanted.

I went into the courtroom when his case was called up, and I walked to the front of the court. The judge asked me who I was and what it was that I wanted. I explained that I was his counselor, and I wanted to say something. The judge asked the defense lawyer if she wanted me to speak and she said no. The judge said she was interested in what I had to say. I explained that I did not believe that this young man should be in this courtroom, but he should be in mental health court. When she looked over at him, he was acting quite strangely, and she looked back at me and stated that she agreed and adjourned him to mental health court. This lawyer was not acting in his best interests, and she had no right not to do so. It was easier for her to have him plead in regular court than have him in Mental Health Court.

I called the detention center regularly because the Ombudsmen's report had been released on the detention center, stating that there had been a lot of cases where people with mental illness in the jail had been beaten up by the guards. I called to make sure that they knew that someone was keeping an eye on this young man while he was incarcerated. I worried that his fatalistic view on life would cause him to encourage an attack. I was able to visit him face to face in a room so I could see whether he was being hurt by anyone. This young man was also part black, so I was also worried about discrimination.

There was also a time when he was taken to the emergency room at one of the hospitals, and when I arrived, I was told he was out of control, and I couldn't see him. I insisted that they let me see him because he knew me, and perhaps he would calm down if he saw me. When I saw him, they had him in a room with a security person at the door.

When I walked in, I just told him it was OK and he could sit down, and he did. I wondered how a hospital could not manage to just be kind to him. When the psychiatrist showed up, she concluded that there was nothing mentally wrong with him and that he was antisocial and just belonged in jail.

She spent about ten minutes with him, if even that. This boy was not antisocial. He did not belong in jail. I worked with him for over two years. I was never at risk with him. He never missed an appointment with me. He had a form of autism, and he had experienced a great deal of rejection by his peers. He had been abandoned by his father as a young child when it was discovered he had autism.

This is not to say we never argued because, yes, we did, and he needed to do that too. Once, he threw a chair and got up to leave, and I said, 'Pick up the chair, put it back and sit down,' and he did. I never feared him, not once.

I had him "formed" by the Justice of the Peace at one point, hoping to get him some professional help and requested that he not be directed to the previous hospital, which had deemed him antisocial. He was not admitted to the new hospital because they stated his issues were too complex. Too complex for whom? What did that mean? Was he not worth helping? Do they only help people with simple problems? Who helps people with more complex problems? Apparently, no one. Even my own agency told me to stop seeing him. Does this not seem crazy? We have a young man, and he can't get professional help because his issues are too complex. What is supposed to happen to him?

I worked with this young man over a two-and-a-half-year period, and he recovered, but not with the help of any of the people who are paid to work with difficult cases. I will tell you that he became a fine young man. He began eating very healthily and doing yoga daily. He would always have difficulty because of the autism piece, but that has more to do with other people than to do with him. I really liked this young man. There was one point in an appointment when I saw him cross the threshold to become a man, and that moment was so unbelievably touching. I was gifted by having the honor to accompany him for that part of his journey, and I have seen him years later and he turned into a kind and generous young man. He could so easily have died in the callous and uncaring world of services to people who are so ready to dispose of people they deem too difficult to treat.

One thing that I saw from early on working with addicted people is that if they had a mental health problem, you could not get them professional help. We were forced to do whatever we could to help our clients because we couldn't find anyone willing to work with them. Many had very serious trauma issues, but no one wanted to work with them.

It wouldn't be until much later that the mental health world would look at concurrent disorders, and then only when the funding dollars were attached to doing that. Even when this happened, you would see inadequate services that never really offered the level of services that people really needed. They would supply only what looked like Concurrent Disorders Services. This would amount to Cognitive Behavioral Therapy and Dialectical Behavioral Therapy groups. One would focus on changing thoughts while the other would focus on emotional regulation and meditation.

It was deemed that emotional regulation was all that was needed. This forced me to work very hard at getting additional education because there was nothing else to do. Unfortunately, we would never make the money that these other people would. We were considered low on qualifications, and certainly I think that was true early on, but time forced many people to elevate their educational backgrounds to meet their clients' needs. There were no other options.

While I worked in the schools, I worked with a fourteen-year-old girl. She had a history of serious sexual abuse issues and was addicted to crack cocaine. At the time I met her, she was using in the evenings with a fifty-two-year-old man who was selling her for sex while providing her with drugs. I sat at a table where the other people included the police, the Children's Aid Society, a psychologist, the principal, a social worker and her mother. Her mother wanted her to be taken into care, but the team decided that was not necessary. The Children's Aid Society stated that she would soon be sixteen, so there was no point in intervening.

I could not understand this at all. These were all the right people sitting around the table agreeing to allow the worst situation to continue, one that anyone should know would have deadly consequences. I left this position shortly afterward because I could not continue to work in a system that thought that this was in any way OK. I also believed that this girl would end up dead without serious intervention or be pulled into some human trafficking situation.

Two years later, I was informed that she had been found dead in a ditch. When the people paid to care about our children deem that it is not necessary to intervene with a child, who is being pimped out by a fifty-two-year-old pedophile in the evening for drugs and is coming to school and sleeping through the day, then I am not willing to stand by and be part of that system. This does not eliminate the fact that you accumulate this tragedy internally. It becomes part of your trauma. One more position of powerlessness where you get to stand by while this society deems that it is OK to let a fourteen-year-old girl be thrown away because she'll be sixteen eventually and, after all, she's already damaged goods.

I had another client who was a fourteen-year-old boy.

You can't imagine sometimes how small a fourteen-year-old is. This guy was so small. He was somewhat lost. His parents had separated and remarried and started new families, and that can leave you feeling like whatever you were part of just doesn't exist anymore. He was very sweet. Then something happened

When I looked at all of the material I had access to, it added up to what looked like a sexual assault by a number of older students in the school. These older guys had been put in the position of mentors over the younger students. They were grade 12 students. This kid had spent a night at one of their places where a number of the other mentors were present. After this he tried to kill himself in a very serious way. That he survived was a miracle and not without serious medical intervention. I had enough material to more than suggest that something serious had happened between the older boys and this kid the night he slept over. A lot of this was on their Facebook interactions. I went to the school psychologist to see what he thought of some of what I had, and he agreed that something did not seem right. I went to the principal of the school, and he determined that in future they might need to be more careful when choosing their mentors. That was it.

I went to my supervisor at my work, and he chose to take no action. I went back to him because I could not see how no one was willing to take any action. He again took no action, but I was told that the student was going to go to a new school, so he would be transferred to a new counselor. I explained that both the mother and the child had wanted me to continue seeing him, but I was told that I wasn't being given a choice and was actually asked if I was choosing to defy their authority. It was clear that they had no intention of dealing with this issue.

Sometime later a new director took over my agency, and

I was now at a new school when I received a call demanding that I return to my agency immediately because the new director wanted to see me. I remember wondering what this was about when I began to think about this case. It was the only thing I could think of that could have any significance or any seriousness that would have someone demand my presence with such an air of emergency.

I had documented this case in great detail in my notes because I wanted to make sure that all this information was on file should anything ever come up concerning this student again. When I got there, she asked me if I had wondered why I was being called in. I said I had thought about it and that case had come to mind. She congratulated me on my documentation and said she had rarely seen someone document something so carefully. I said that I found the whole thing rather upsetting, so I felt it needed to be documented since it had not been dealt with, and I had been removed from the client's care. She asked me why. The two managers that had done that were sitting there and I pointed to them and said they removed me. They said they didn't know about what had gone on and I cut them off and said, "You knew everything because I made it very clear what had gone on. You still chose to remove the student, despite the fact that the mother asked me to continue with her son and that he had asked to continue to see me." She thanked me for my work and let me go.

I thought that now it would be dealt with. Interestingly one week later, she was walked out of the building and out of her job. She had been fired. Now what was that all about? Is there some sort of agreement that we don't deal with the sexual abuse of children? This took place somewhere in 2010 or later. The school covered it up, and my agency covered it up. A kid almost died. That is very disturbing to me.

I have never understood some of the responses I saw around things like this. In this case I wondered whether one of the mentors wasn't someone from an important family, and that's why it just didn't matter but I don't really know. It's possible, because the kid that was impacted wasn't from a prominent family. I think there has to be a reason why because, if not, there is something seriously wrong in our world. But I would see things that seriously disturbed me over and over again in the agencies I worked in. I would be targeted by them as well. In the end I chose not to return to the addiction field because there were just too many seriously unwell people working there. I have said that working in the addiction field caused me a moral injury that was traumatic. I saw things that I had a hard time living with. I am still haunted by many of them.

I will mention that there were people who worked in addiction agencies at various levels who relapsed into their addiction and continued to work after having relapsed and died as a result. Some of these incidents were very traumatic for the clients that were involved with them. That might be an argument for not having recovering people in the field, but I have also heard stories about non-identified people who are every bit as ill working in the field. I worked for one agency where I was doing some part time work and then chose to leave when COVID prevented outside people from going in. I was later informed by staff there that I had been fired after I had physically beaten up the director while drunk at a party. I thought that was interesting since I don't go to parties nor drink and have rarely ever seen the director, not to mention the fact that I don't beat people up. This story was apparently coming from the director and all I could think of was this person had to be rather unwell because there just seemed to be no reason to come up with this story. I had left under no negative circumstances and had no negative interactions with this woman. Why did she need to tell this story? What was she afraid of? I do know that there were some unhealthy things going on there, but I could not have verified much of that, so I posed no real threat to her.

I saw things happening around me that were not in my workplace, that also made me wonder. I remember once being downtown on Rideau Street and I was walking to the bus stop when I heard a girl crying behind me. She was saying, "I just want to go home," over and over. I turned around because it was disturbing, and I saw a very young girl with a guy in his mid-twenties. He was saying, "Stop it, I'll get you a bottle." She said she wanted to call her mother, and he said he would call her, and he had a phone in his hand. He had a hold of her, and they went just behind some construction boards near the bus stop. At one point I saw her on her knees pleading with him.

I thought it looked an awful lot like a human trafficking situation. I asked her if she needed help, and she shook her head no. I decided to call 911. I described what I had seen and the fact that they were still there. They sent the mall security out just to make sure that they didn't leave. I stayed in case they needed me to tell them what I had seen.

The police showed up and went to talk to them. They did not separate the two people but talked to them together. The police came out from behind the boards laughing and walked away. I couldn't believe it. Why hadn't they done more?

The girl looked to be about thirteen or fourteen years old. She was dressed in a way that didn't look like she was street savvy. She had said she wanted to go home. All they had to do was say they were taking her home because there seemed to be some problem with them, and if there wasn't she could always come back.

I called the police the next day to report the situation and ask them to explain why they had not separated the two people to talk to them. They said that not all the police were trained on how to deal with potential human trafficking situations. I don't think that separating them to have a conversation would have been rocket science, and I don't believe that they wouldn't have known that.

The question remains as to why this wasn't important enough that they chose not to intervene, given that we do have a human trafficking problem in the city, and the long-term psychological damage caused by these experiences is very serious. As far as the officers not being trained, it wasn't hard to get, since I had managed to get both online education and in-person training with very little effort.

So just what is it? Is it just not worth it? Is it just too much trouble? Are our children just not worth that much that we can't drive them home just to be on the safe side? There's another face I won't forget.

Youth were also being impacted by opiate overdoses very early on in what would become an epidemic. In one summer, four young people that I was connected to died. It was devastating. When you work with young people, you can quickly see all the potential they have within them. When they die as young people it is devastating. I had done some research at that point on what, if anything, we could have done to help these young people. I came across Naloxone kits in the United States, and I thought that this seemed like a good idea. It would be another five years before this became a viable and available tool in our city. The situation had to get grave enough to cause a reaction because, after all, if people were dying from opiates, they were taking them themselves.

I feel like I have been fighting for people who have lost their significance as people. It doesn't matter who they are or who they are important to, their drug or alcohol use disqualifies them for our serious concern. I remember one young man in the schools telling me about his friend who had died from being stabbed to death in the market. I told him that we, as a society, did not know who we had lost. This young man might have gone on to become a person that we needed in the world, but now we would never know who we had lost. I said the same to him. I said we cannot afford to lose you either because we do not know who you will be, and we may need you too. He was significant, as are all individuals, especially if we treat them as such.

Over and over, I have asked myself why we are not responding to the call for compassion and intervention. How many generations will pay the price for our inadequate responses? Our current response to addiction says it all. Let's just leave them in their addiction as if that's a place where we should leave anyone. Having been there, I can assure you that's a hell you should never condemn anyone to. But I believe that the government has a more sinister goal in mind, but I will get to that later.

It is also important to speak about our schools, where we do next to nothing to teach our children to stop hurting each other. I saw a constant "look the other way" policy in the schools, because there was nothing in place to change the attitude of kids who helped themselves feel better by putting someone else down. Their education needs to include how to be decent to each other. We need to ask where their anger is coming from and help them with that. Despite the services available, the problem persists. The education on how to be caring has to start from day one. We cannot let one day go by without stressing the need to be compassionate and caring people. We have to nurture kindness in every single school our children attend.

The pain of rejection breeds drug addiction. It is the one place where you can guarantee to find acceptance when everyone else has rejected you. The only admission criteria for this group are a willingness to use drugs or alcohol. It changes the game. I went from absolutely isolated to part of the minute

I started drinking alcohol underage. Drug use increased my acceptance.

When I was working with youth, I recognized very quickly that I had to gain their trust, and my age was so distant from them that it would be hard for them to be able to believe that I could relate to them or understand them.

I have always believed that the way to create connection is common ground, and the way I saw it rap music was something they seemed to relate to. I spent about six months walking around listening to Tupac. I asked my nephew who I should be listening to if I wanted to learn about rap music, and he gave me six Tupac CDs. It took a while to be able to catch the lyrics and the style, but I have always loved music, so I was willing to give this a try. I also thought the lyrics might tell me something about what held meaning for them. I grew to like Tupac and, after watching a film called "Thug Angel," I really saw how very talented and bright this young man had been.

I have been a poet for most of my life and I could really appreciate their ability to rhyme. I have always been a rhyming poet and some of these rap performers could really rhyme. In fact, they taught me a lot more about ways to rhyme than I had ever known. Eminem is incredibly talented and innovative when it comes to rhyme. It wasn't hard for me to become interested in this genre, although some of the messaging was very concerning to me. I thought, if kids are listening to this then they are getting a pro-drug, pro-gang and pro-violence message. It was troubling enough for me to want to do something about it.

After listening to enough rap, it began to really change the way I wrote poetry. I realized I liked the rhythmic style of rap, and I began to write in that format. It wasn't long before I became interested in how these guys made their music. A lot of kids dream of being big rap stars, and so a lot of the kids I met made beats and wrote raps. It didn't take me long to do research to find out how to do this. I bought a music program and got my hands on some music loops and gave it a try. Then I got a good microphone and began to record my poetry and then added some music to it. The next step was to figure out how to make a video and lay the music track on it. I decided to have it play against a pencil drawing related to the subject matter of the poem. I began doing drawings that would be specifically related to the poems I was writing.

My first rap had a chorus that said, "All you kids need to pull your heads from the crapper, because all you've been listening to is another lame rapper." It was part of the style to be a sort of back-and-forth challenge, and this one attacked the over focus on some of the language, sexism and drug money messages. If I was going to get into the conversation with them, I needed to say it in a way where they would pay attention. I uploaded a number of these to YouTube, and when I had a youth who gave me one of those, "What could you possibly know about anything," attitudes, I gave them a link and asked them to check it out.

I also saw that many rappers spoke about the difficulties they had with their mothers or their fathers. It seemed like they were using their poetry to try and deal with the difficulties they had experienced in their lives. Eminem had written a lot about his mother, and over the years he had changed how he saw her, and he had softened his message. You could see how he matured over time. J. Cole and Yellow Wolf both spoke about their absent fathers. There was some real relevance to some of this music's attraction to youth. It not only provided them with a voice, but it spoke directly to some of their most painful issues. I could see its importance, and I could use it to open discussions with the youth.

I eventually created a classroom presentation on the messages from rap music and the therapeutic use of rap. I used three examples from rap and one that I wrote. I encouraged youth to try the genre as a way of speaking about themselves and their own story. This was very successful with the kids.

It worked! I was in. It really changed things with the kids, and I'm sure the fact that I went to that length to relate to them didn't go amiss. I put up a Tupac poster and a Bob Marley poster in my office, and that worked as well. Some kids showed up just to see the posters. I also had the distinction of having seen Bob Marley in concert. The kids taught me a lot. And I have always realized that if you're going to reach someone, you have to walk a little distance into their world before they can be sure you actually give a damn. The beauty of doing this is you may walk away with something you hadn't expected to get in return. In all my time working with kids I got as much from them as I may have given them in return.

There was one boy who was from another country. He had been in Canada for maybe three or four years. He lost his sister to a medical issue when he was only four years old. He had loved her dearly and they had been close. They had always looked at the moon together. It was difficult for him when she died because his parents were grieving and weren't able to attend to his grief. I realized that he needed to have someone witness his grief.

I wrote a poem about the story of their relationship and everything he had told me about that time in his life. I knew that there had been a musician who wrote a song about looking at the moon I just had to figure out who it was. I finally found it. It was "Talking to The Moon" by Don Henley from The Eagles. It was a beautiful piano piece. It took me a while to set up the music so I could take the lyrics out except for the chorus and lay my poem in place of them. Then I printed a CD with a picture of the moon with the title "Children of the Moon." I also printed out a full picture of the moon with the lyrics printed on top. He had said he had wanted a picture of the moon, but he could never take a good one. I had taken many.

The next time I saw him I told him I had something that I wanted him to hear, and I had my headphones on me, and the song was on an iPod. I put them on him and pushed play. I watched him listen and I watched the tears fall down his face. I witnessed his grief, and the poem told him that I had heard him. It was such a beautiful moment. I gave him both the CD and the picture afterwards. It was such a privilege to be able to do that for him. He was such a beautiful young man, and he had such a beautiful heart.

One young boy came to my office once just to see the posters I had. I invited him in. He began to talk about himself. He was concerned about his own behavior, and he was holding himself accountable. He was hanging around some pretty rough guys, and it sounded like they were trying to pull him into a gang. He didn't like some of the things he had been doing with them. He would talk about the things that bothered him, and then he would leave. He would come back repeatedly, talking through the things that he was struggling with. He talked about wanting to be a clothing designer. I bought him a sketch pad and some pencils so he could do some designs. He started drawing some designs and he was good. He was such an interesting young man. He got a job through the school as a job placement, and when he got his first paycheck, he bought his grandmother $100.00 worth of groceries. He lived with her because his own mother didn't want to take care of him. You could see what he had to struggle with at such a young age. He lived in a poor area of the city where there was a lot of pull from the gangs. What amazed me was the depth of his thinking. He wrestled with his thoughts about right and wrong and how he could see that those in the gangs crossed over to a place where they lost some aspect of their humanity. He was only fifteen, yet he had the capacity to consider these things despite the limitations of his circumstances. I felt honored to have the privilege of being the person he had chosen to share his thoughts with.

There were so many times when I found myself really blessed to be in the position to accompany many young people through some very difficult periods in their lives. I will never forget how difficult it was for me as a young person. I knew how profound young people could be. I considered it a gift to be able to be there for them. When they were able to trust me and be open, I was very touched by that. I cared very deeply for them. To be given the opportunity to come into the lives of young people and, for a brief time, offer some support is a very special thing. I wanted to be able to give them that sense that they were special and that their lives were important. Adolescence is such a very difficult time for some young people. I wanted to make sure that those who were struggling knew that someone cared.

Your Best Intentions Might Get You Nowhere

I took counseling seriously, and anyone who knows me knows that about me. I will fight for my clients. I will go beyond what most people would do. I will try and get all the referrals, and I will persist in trying to get what they need to be successful. If I don't know about the issue they are dealing with, I will find out about it.

When faced with a client with a brain injury, I took a brain injury course at some financial cost to myself. I knew that if I was going to be successful working with him, I needed to know how he had been affected by that injury. He was in a court program, and he would not be able to meet the same expectations as the other clients due to that injury. I needed to be able to explain that to the court team. He also needed to be seen by a brain injury clinic to see what was happening to his brain since he had not had any follow-up since his initial operation after the injury that had taken place over a year earlier. I went through the process of arranging a referral for him and also looked into other resources that might be available to him.

I also suspected that he had Asperger's or some form of high-functioning autism. After meeting his father on one occasion, I became sure that he had autism because his father had the same presentation. This client's drug use came about because he was alienated from his peers as a young person in school. He revealed that he was seen as different by his peers and that this caused him a great deal of anxiety. He found that taking opiates relieved this. This led to long-term substance abuse. He was never identified as having autism. I gave him a long questionnaire on autism and asked him to go through it and tell me if he resonated with any of the items on the questionnaire. He returned it and told me that it all made sense to him, and he wondered why no one had ever said anything to him.

I wondered if we could have avoided the seriousness of his addiction if someone might have identified what was going on with him and been able to help all those years ago. By the time I met him he was addicted to opiates, amphetamines, and benzodiazepines. He was on the government's golden trio of drugs, and we couldn't get him off of them. They were all being prescribed to him by this point. There's no incentive to stop using drugs when the government is willing to supply them to you.

Education was an important part of my job. I never relied on whether the agency I worked for would pay for my training because addiction agencies are chronically underfunded. I paid for, about 97% of all the training that I have taken over the years, and a list of courses I have taken spans seven typed pages. As someone who was expected to help people, I knew I needed to be knowledgeable and if I wasn't, then I needed to become that. I needed to know what the problem was and then how or who could address it. None of this is easy because I found myself up against many professionals who would not open the door.

The interesting thing about professionals and other agencies is their absolute arrogance. My best description would be to say that not many agencies play nice in the sandbox. You would almost have to prostrate yourself to them and even then, you'd be lucky if they would even see your client. I have no idea what this is all about. I don't know how many times I have seen professionals dismissing clients for completely unknown reasons. It would be like playing the lottery if you could get someone seen and that didn't mean much because that didn't guarantee they would get services.

I remember going through all the paperwork to refer this one guy to treatment, and he finally got a telephone interview only to find out he needed to go to treatment before being able to go to their treatment center. This all took weeks to do this work, and if you had known that you wouldn't have bothered. You would have just tried another treatment center. If you wonder why people don't make it, I could give you hundreds of reasons why, and they wouldn't be about the person.

I met a guy who had a very serious alcohol addiction, and he had gone to see a doctor for some help. The doctor prescribed him benzodiazepines, knowing if the guy just tried to stop, he could have a seizure and be at risk of dying. The man knew nothing about meds or drugs. He had never tried to stop drinking before. He took the pills while drinking and ended up pouring some boiling water down his leg and injuring his shoulder. He went to the hospital who bandaged up the burns and sent him home. I saw him about a day later. He was wearing shorts, and the bandage on his leg wasn't in place. His burns looked horrible. He reported that his shoulder was really bothering him as well, and he showed a very discolored shoulder. He had mentioned this at the hospital, but they did not really give it much of a look.

I called to see if I could get him into a medical detox for alcohol and benzos, but he required a referral from the hospital, and they had not been willing to do that. His family and I finally found a detox out of town, and he went. While he was there, they had his shoulder looked at and discovered it was broken. It was two weeks after being seen at the emergency department of the hospital. The problem was that he was intoxicated at the hospital, and that made him not worth treating. This was not an aggressive man when drunk, so that would not have been a reason. This is the problem that I have seen happen repeatedly in the prescribing of benzodiazepines to people with severe alcoholism, who are then left to go home and take them unsupervised. These drugs are extremely similar to alcohol, which is why they are used to detoxify people who have severe alcoholism.

Alcohol and Benzodiazepines are the only two drugs where you can die from the withdrawal. In a medical detox, which is required if you are going to stop either of these drugs, you are given doses of benzos, which are lowered slowly over time. Giving someone with serious alcoholism these drugs and sending them home is dangerous. Too much can stop the respiratory system, put you in a coma and kill you. It's highly irresponsible to expect that a person with a serious alcohol addiction would be able to manage detoxing themselves with benzos safely. There are medical advisory reports that state that you do not prescribe these to people with addiction.

I was at a Primary Care Convention once, and a woman who had a very prestigious job in medical education gave a talk. She used a case example where she had a patient who had relapsed to her drinking, and she gave her a prescription for benzodiazepines to come off the alcohol. The woman died. I asked her later why she had given her that prescription rather than having her go to a medical detox. The woman did not appreciate my question and brushed me off. I later sent her an e-mail, and when she replied she admitted that, yes, the woman should have been sent to a medical detox. She'd made a mistake. Oh well, too bad for the woman. I had been insistent on addressing this because the week before I had just lost a friend that I had known for over twenty years for this very reason. In his case he was prescribed benzodiazepines and relapsed to alcohol and then killed himself very violently. The institution that prescribed the meds to him had access to his file that detailed a serious past alcohol addiction.

I knew this man from attending twelve-step meetings for

over twenty years. We attended the same discussion group every week. I knew him personally and we talked many times. He was a very tortured soul. He had a horrific childhood, and it had taken a terrible toll on his mental health. He was haunted. It hurt me to see him that way because he deserved better. I told him one time to come to a lecture on PTSD that was being given at a mental health hospital. Maybe they would have some suggestions on how to help him. He was courageous enough to go to the microphone and ask where he could get some help. The speaker was kind enough to speak to him afterwards and worked in the hospital and agreed to see him. I thought finally he would get the help he needed.

Over the next few weeks, he didn't look like he was getting better but worse. I spoke to him, and he said they had given him some medications, including benzodiazepines. I was confused about why they would do that because he had a severe history of addiction, which included almost dying from cirrhosis. They would have had a record of this because he had been seen by the hospital before related to his addiction. A week later, we received word that he had killed himself. His family stated that he had returned to drinking and then decided to slit his own throat. That was devastating to me. I was so angry that I wrote to the CEO of the hospital to complain. They never wrote me back.

I sent a very angry e-mail to the doctor who had agreed to see him. He wrote back asking me why I was so angry at him. I said that he should never have been prescribed benzodiazepines in the first place. I told him I was angry because he had the power to do something about this practice because he had the credentials, but no one ever takes the actions that they should, and people keep dying as a result.

To his credit, he did reach out to me and said he had brought the issue up with the hospital, but again a good man was dead. This man had a daughter. He didn't need to die that way. This is a mental health hospital that supposedly has knowledge of addiction, so how the hell does this even happen? It happens because of arrogance. It happened because people get to say Addiction and Mental Health as if that is true when it is not.

The words Addiction and Mental Health began to be bandied about when they became popular as words sometimes become. It's like the flavor of the month. At one point, the addiction was to be treated first before the mental health condition could be looked at, but then that changed, and it was thought that both should be taken care of. This made it sound like somehow psychiatry and addiction experts would be working together. This couldn't be further from the truth. The two had no intention of having anything to do with each other. The addiction people could treat the addiction, and psychiatry would look at the mental health issues and never shall the two meet, and that's how things were. Whatever they sold to the public was not what was going on in reality. That was the secret they had no intention of revealing.

This meant that psychiatry could prescribe something that addiction would not agree was a good idea, say benzodiazepines, for example. Addiction would tell the client they could not take that medication, but when they went back to psychiatry, they were told to take it. Even though the two disciplines were in the same organization, one would not pick up the phone and talk to the other. This left the client trying to figure out what to do. When I confronted the head doctor from the addiction unit at a conference about this just after she claimed that the two groups worked hand in hand, she told me if I had a complaint I should file it.

In hospitals the lines were clearly drawn. Addictions were in one place, and Mental health was in another. In other agencies, mental health agencies invited addiction counselors into their groups to participate. The marriage was not as consensual as it would seem, and they had no intention of getting into bed with each other.

Eventually, the mental health hospital decided to dispense with all of its Addiction Counselors and replace them with Social Workers. I think this sent a very strong message about the addiction field that went something like this: This field was never legitimate, it never had any real qualifications, and now that addiction would be viewed as a concurrent disorder that would be seen as best treated with Cognitive Behavioral Therapy and Dialectical Behavioral Therapy for emotional regulation and less focused on the substance abuse issue Addiction Counselors would be unnecessary. They were, in fact, what was seen as relics of a best-forgotten paradigm. So they would treat people with a substance abuse issue without any reference to the substance they were using or the effects of this substance or its withdrawal.

This was in keeping with the government's support of harm reduction and the legalization of marijuana. There were a lot of changes coming up. To those of us still working with addiction, this was disturbing. Unfortunately, a lot of changes were also happening in the agencies. The hiring of social workers had been going on for some time, which meant that there were more and more people who had less personal knowledge of addiction in the field. We began to see more educated people, but they didn't necessarily have education in the area of addiction. The wages for working in addiction were still very low in the agencies. The highest wage for most of the years I worked in the field was $19.00 an hour. At the very end we had managed to get $26.00 an hour at my agency when we had become unionized.

I think what was getting to me was that I was trying to address all of these issues, but only the people with the credentials were considered knowledgeable enough to address them, and they didn't seem to really care about it. To this day, benzodiazepines are overprescribed to already addicted people. The current trend in harm reduction seems to be to prescribe people on methadone benzodiazepines, which, if you check the literature, is contraindicated. They are both sedating to the central nervous system and can cause death. I have seen a person OD, and when they administered Naloxone, they didn't come out of it because they were also overdosing on benzodiazepines, which don't respond to Naloxone. I believe this is part of a new trend related loosely to the Harm Reduction efforts, which has decided to provide addicted people with amphetamines and benzodiazepines along with methadone or Dilaudid because they were abusing all of these drugs initially.

Everyone points to Portugal as having used this idea to deal with their country's drug abuse problem. Portugal decriminalized drug abuse. They did not legalize it or provide the drugs. They reduced their police response to the problem, which had been 90% of their financial investment, while 10% had been in treatment. They reversed this by putting 90% of their expenditure into treatment. People were no longer charged with their use, but they were diverted to a commission that recommended treatment options and provided sanctions when their recommendations weren't followed. The focus on treatment is what produced the promising results in Portugal, not the decriminalization per se. People tend to say that Portugal legalized drug use and this changed the situation, but this is not true.

The problem in this country is that we are unwilling to put the money into effective treatment, and so the claim is made that we must wait until the addicted person chooses to want to change. Anyone who has worked with people with addiction knows that making a choice while you are addicted is like trying to walk an obstacle course while you are blind.

This pretense of respecting the person's right to make a choice is just a very effective way of allowing addiction to continue.

There are monetary benefits to allowing addiction to continue. In Canada, a lot of money is made through legal addictions like cigarettes, alcohol, lottery, gambling, and now pot. The most recent income estimate as of August 2020 for pot is $4.66 billion. When we challenge addiction, we look at all addictions. All of the legal addictions have had a very negative fallout for people who have addiction as an illness. Even though tobacco is the most seriously life-threatening addiction, it has never been eliminated. The taxes have gone up, and the number of smokers has gone down, but it remains an addiction with a high death toll and, with that, a burgeoning weight on our healthcare system. When the government makes financial cuts, they are made to the healthcare system. So, in other words, let's continue to support behaviors that have serious health implications and when a person becomes ill, we can blame them for their unhealthy choices and refuse to support meaningful health responses. Oh, and before I forget, let's tax therapy just in case someone is trying to get well. Never mind the fact that, for most people, therapy is not available because they have no coverage and can't afford it.

I have worked in places that have hired the new staff now considered appropriate for addiction agencies in their attempt to find some legitimacy after years of being deemed unqualified. These people are often social workers or registered psychotherapists with no background in addiction and often haven't a clue how to deal with people who have addiction issues. They often have no idea how different substances affect people. There is an entire neuroscience to how drugs and alcohol affect the brain of a person both during and after they use. This has a significant impact on their ability to function. The effects can be present up to two or more years after the person has stopped their use.

Head injuries are often common in this group, as well as mental health disorders. These clients are often rather complex because they will also often have a history of trauma. It is not unusual to see people on the spectrum for autism. These complexities are the common presentation rather than the exception. People working with addictions had to find a way to deal with this because no one wanted to work with these clients. We had to get educated because we had no other choice, and granted, many people probably didn't take things as seriously as I did, but I'm sure that some people did and got some relevant education to manage some of this. I was able to qualify to become a registered psychotherapist, but I had to leave the addiction field in order to be paid a reasonable salary and to avoid working for unethical people.

Another trend offered by methadone clinics is prescription amphetamines and benzodiazepines since their clients also consume these drugs along with their opiates. Their mantra is recovery your way or, perhaps better put, no recovery at all. They were kindly providing the amphetamines that were landing my client in emergency psychiatric facilities for severe psychosis that had him convinced that his neighbors were bugging his apartment with the intent to kill him. It is unlikely that he will ever recover because of the number of drugs he gets prescribed to him, and the complications caused by a serious brain injury and autism. It is more likely that he will die from his use or the consequences of his use.

We have been in the midst of a Pandemic. COVID-19 has forced an economic shutdown, and people have been instructed to stay socially distant from each other. It is clear that, in order to safeguard the health of the country, certain measures have to be taken. There are currently consequences for contravening these guidelines. We do this because one person does not have the right to engage in behaviors that endanger others. Addiction is one of these behaviors that endangers and harms others. When we give the addicted person a choice, we remove the choices of others. If addiction only harms the person who is using the drugs, then the choice argument makes sense. But even then, when that person's choices cost a huge amount to provide medical care for issues that arise from the person's use, what should we say or do?

It would be significant to point out that the safeguards for COVID did not apply to people who were addicted as I had to travel through the areas they lived in and frequented, and they were not required to wear masks on buses nor even pay the fare for that matter. I point this out since I contracted COVID on the buses despite wearing a mask. I believe this was directly related to the many intoxicated people who got on the buses and fell all over other people while not wearing a mask. I contracted COVID before the vaccines, and this resulted in developing COPD despite the fact that I do not smoke. I have had long COVID since 2019. This has had a huge impact on my health and the quality of my life. When I reached out to the mayor of my city, I was told that these people could not be compelled to wear masks on the bus.

I was raised in an addicted home. If I were to add up the cost of just treating the effect that this had on me as an individual in treatment and in psychiatry, medication, and therapy over the thirty-one years that I have been in recovery, the bill would astound you. The loss of years of a healthy life is the majority of my life, since most of it has been spent trying to get free of the toll that it took on me. Addiction has affected my entire life. Addiction claimed the lives of my parents and many other family members. Addiction carried through the generations of my family. At the age of eighteen, I became parentless, and at a much younger age, I had already lost any sense of family and any family care. My own marriage failed because of addiction. I lost my sister, at the age of fifty-one, to addiction. I chose to have no children because the upbringing I experienced had so negatively affected me I could not risk having children and subjecting them to something similar. My family members died of cancer related to their addiction. Addiction devastated my family and my life. Yet despite the magnitude of addiction's effect, we somehow think we need to let people who are addicted and unable to make a choice have the chance to make a choice they cannot make. This clearly indicates that there is some other agenda operating here. What is somebody gaining from allowing addiction to continue and refusing to fund its treatment? How did harm reduction become the treatment of choice?

The current clinics that offer Methadone also offer Amphetamines, Benzodiazepines and Dilaudid. That covers the range of drugs that the addicted person likes to abuse. It's one-stop shopping, but it doesn't stop them from buying drugs from the street. It's the part of addiction those who have never been addicted don't get. It's like what you see if you ever go into one of the housing units, provided the people deemed unable to manage their own housing. I remember asking someone who worked there if they would take their dog there, and she said no. There was a good reason for that. It's not something they'll ever show you pictures of, but someone should take a camera into these places, and we can all have a look at how compassionate we're all being. You might want to wear a hazmat suit though. It kind of looks like some third-world hell hole. People are living in their own filth.

When check day arrives, it gets really scary. You might arrive to see people crawling across the floor, but don't be alarmed, it's all part of the ambiance. We should all be relieved that they are being taken care of. This is where addiction becomes the ugliest, but somehow, we're told that this is a great service we're doing. I do not accept that this is in any way an acceptable way to treat human beings. Some may call this harm reduction, but I call it a travesty, an absolute criminal action.

No human being should ever be left in these conditions in a country such as ours. We should hang our heads in shame, and one day this will come to light, and we will have to live with the shame of allowing it to have ever taken place. We will never be able to come up with an excuse for this, and nothing we say will ever explain it. It will be one more story of inhumanity that this country will have to bear, and just how many people's names will be added to the list of the dead. The question I would like to ask some of the people who are advocates for Harm Reduction: is that what you would want for your child, your sister or brother, or your mother or father? People can recover. They can have a better quality of life.

I knew one person who had schizophrenia and was also diabetic. He had the luxury of harm reduction. When I first met him, he was in the 12 step rooms, and he had all of his limbs, but after he started with Harm Reduction, he started to lose his limbs. He had several procedures to have parts of his legs amputated and I was wondering how much of him he would have to lose before they might consider that harm reduction might not be working for him.

As far as providing drugs to addicts, what the Harm Reduction people don't understand is that people will still use street drugs because there is never enough. People use to escape, and sometimes they just continue to use until they are completely gone. Sometimes the goal is Russian Roulette. The depth of addiction is not a happy place. You have to be there to understand that and having been there I know what it felt like. It was a trap that was almost impossible to get out of and sometimes you just used without caring how far you went, because in that mental state, it really didn't matter.

I know I became careless with my life because my life ceased to have much meaning after a while. I took chances with the drugs I used, with the amounts and the combinations. I often wondered why they didn't kill me, and I often didn't care if they had. There were many times I was disappointed that they didn't, but it wasn't like I was telling people about that. That's just how I felt. It's why someone gets their methadone, then scores some fentanyl, goes home and does it and dies. It's not an accident. You think you're doing them this big favor by giving them their drugs, like that's this big kindness when the addiction is the hell in which they're caught. You give them no hope, just the hell, because by that point the drugs don't work anymore, and that's why death becomes the game.

You don't get it, and that's why you make me so damn mad. Your good intentions do nothing but harm. You could offer them a way out of hell, but instead you offer them a way to fall further in, and you will never get that. You will stand there self-righteously, like you have the right answers, and look at people like me, like somehow, I don't understand and don't really care. But I want these people to really have a life, not the shitty existence that you think is all they should have, because somehow you think they are choosing that hell. So really, which one of us is twisted?

They are caught in a trap that owns them, and they cannot see their way out. So instead of helping them find a way out, you help them stay trapped and you think that's kindness. You ask them what they want when they can only have one answer because they are addicted. They cannot imagine anything else from the place where they are. It's simpler to just appease their addiction than to help ignite some hope for something better. You can pat yourself on the back and say I gave them what they wanted. It's not my problem if they choose something that destroys them. At least I was trying to keep them alive. And there it is. Let's do as little as possible.

It has recently been recognized that bringing people back

from an overdose does not save them from the brain damage they experience during the period when they have overdosed and before the Naloxone takes effect. So, we may be saving their lives, but each overdose is causing more and more damage to their brain, affecting their mental capacity. So, I will ask again: how much harm reduction are we actually doing?

After having worked for twenty-seven years in the field of addiction, all I have learned is how we lack the value of the lives of people who have fallen into addiction. When the social system fails to protect children, and believe me it does, these children suffer, and there is nothing in place to help them. It is cheaper and easier to gain access to drugs and alcohol than it is to get mental health help. When poverty is impossible to escape you may as well drink away the little you have because at least you can escape for a bit. When those in strategic positions turn their heads when wrong things take place and refuse to act, and believe me, they do, children are left as victims over and over again. When hospitals refuse to treat those in need but throw people out of the doors of their hospitals because they are addicted, where do they go but back to the streets? When parents come in through those doors with their children, only to be told their child is an addict and there is nothing they are prepared to do to help, what does that parent do? When doctors prescribe benzodiazepines over and over to people who are addicted, knowing that these drugs are addictive, they end up with a problem no one wants to treat.

How many times do sexual abuse situations arise in places where they should not be taking place, and all of the people who should be looking out for our children do absolutely nothing when they have been notified but choose to hide it instead? I'm not pulling these things out of the air; they have all happened and I have been there trying to get the right people to take action to no avail.

How does a mental health hospital kick a young person

out of their hospital because they tried to kill themselves while they were there? They then ended up killing themselves. How does a nurse in a hospital think it is in any way ethical to throw things at a young man in a bed who has lost feeling in his body to see if his feeling has come back, purely because he disclosed that he had smoked a joint? Tell me that you agree with me that these things make no sense. Tell me that you, too, find this stuff appalling. You cannot believe that any of this is OK.

I spoke with a mother whose twenty-one-year-old son died in her arms before the paramedics got there and were able to revive him. She was traumatized by that experience. When they got to the hospital, they sat him in a chair and refused to put him in a bed because he was an addict. She was beside herself because she had thought she had lost her son only a short time before. She was asking them to find a bed for him and they were treating her like she was as unimportant as they thought he was. She was shocked and stunned that this was the way they were treating both her and her son.

Sometime later, her son eventually died of an overdose. She never recovered from that. He had been sexually abused as a young boy. He never recovered from that. Can you imagine what pain she was left with after his death?

I knew this young man, and he was a beautiful young man. If you had met him, you would never have known he was addicted to opiates because he just didn't look like he was addicted. I saw her pain, and I will never forget him or her. I never felt so absolutely useless in my life because there was nothing, I could do to help either of them. It's not that he couldn't be helped; it's that we don't live in a country that is willing to help. We failed them.

The stories of the lives of the people that I worked with who were addicted were most often stories of trauma. That they used drugs or alcohol was no surprise. That they couldn't stop using them was also no surprise. There were never enough resources to help them. The resources were never there when they needed them. The waiting lists were too long. There were often too many hoops to jump through, too many restrictions, and for some reason or another, they just couldn't get into whatever place you tried to get them into. Sometimes you sent them somewhere, and they got sicker there than they were before going there.

A lot of times it was the sheer arrogance of the agencies themselves. They acted as gatekeepers to their own little private domains where they had the power over life and death. It's like they never considered that part. They never took into consideration how ill the clients were because if they didn't behave perfectly according to their script, they would find themselves back out the door or simply crossed off the list altogether.

Heaven forbids you showed up to an addiction and mental health facility and showed any signs that you weren't mentally well. That would get you ejected pretty quickly. You may have been raised in the wild, but you had better have figured out how to civilize yourself before asking for help, because otherwise you weren't going to get any help. Some of these places treated their clients abusively.

The Magic of Language

All along, the pendulum swung back and forth on how negative or positive addicted people were being viewed. There was a lot of money to be made on ideas of how we could destigmatize addiction, and most of that centered on language. The idea being that if we changed the language, we used to refer to addicted people, suddenly people's attitudes would change.

I like to refer to this as the linguistic sleight of hand. Now you see it, now you don't. The new language was to remove the word addiction because that had a bad connotation to it.

The new words would be substance use, and substance use disorder. This got rid of that nasty idea that people could be addicted and clearly identified drug use as a choice so that people could be allowed to use substances and not be stigmatized by using substances. Now I hope that people can see what this magic language shift just did. If people are no longer addicted and drug use is a choice, then we don't need to do anything about it because it is up to the person whether they want to use substances or not.

This opens the doors to providing them with the drugs that they use, not that this in any way stops the purchase of street drugs because they will still buy street drugs. It reduces the need for treatment because if people are given the message that drug use is a choice that they get to make, chances are they won't choose to stop. They won't choose to stop because they are, in fact, addicted, because changing the language did not change the facts, and this was all a political game in the first place. Meanwhile, this has done nothing whatsoever to reduce the stigma of addiction. Hospitals have exactly the same attitudes, communities still want these people out of their neighborhoods, because, believe me, if you live where they live, it is truly crazy, and most people don't want to treat them.

It seems that regardless of how much more we know about addiction today, it has done nothing to change attitudes towards addiction. One of the things I began to see while I was working in addiction was the appearance of a group of people who showed up with alcoholism that had never had this problem until they had bariatric surgery. I thought this was interesting because it posed a problem for this group. For one, they were very angry. They had never had a problem with alcohol, but once they had the surgery, they seemed to become almost instant alcoholics.

It was rather interesting. Apparently, the surgery, which makes the stomach smaller, also interferes with the processing of alcohol, so that when the person drinks, they are affected by the alcohol sooner so that they become drunk faster. The attraction to alcohol is very much related to why they had surgery in the first place and very related to the understanding of traumas, the reason why people become addicted. The ACE study I mentioned earlier also pointed to obesity as an outcome of trauma, so their initial problem of overeating, that led them to seek help with their weight issues was related to trauma. The doctors did not do anything about the origins of the eating issue but addressed the weight problem through surgery, so that the person was still at risk, and so when they drank it would be predictable that they would develop an alcohol issue. The other predictable outcome we see is that many of these people eventually regain weight over time. Clearly, not addressing the origin of the issue did not result in a successful outcome and, in this case, led to other complications.

I noticed that the counselors where I was working did not understand these clients very well because they did not respond well to their anger. I got it clearly why they were angry. They signed up for surgery, but they had not signed up for alcoholism. These people had become alcoholics through no fault of their own. It was caused by surgery which had interfered with the metabolism of alcohol. They needed to be allowed to work through the anger they felt because it was a righteous anger. They would also have to deal with the grief of no longer being able to drink.

I was always interested in trying to reach out to various places to provide information and I tried many ways to do this. I volunteered my time over and over to hospitals and research groups, trying to get a foot in the door to be able to offer some talks on addiction, both as a professional and as a person of lived experience. I was more than qualified. I had grown up in an addicted family, I had become addicted, I had recovered from addiction, and I had worked in the addiction field for over twenty-seven years. I was an intelligent and well-informed person. I was both passionate and compassionate. I felt that I had a lot to offer. I found out that it is unbelievably hard to get your foot in the door. Most places are happy to have you give your time to do what they want, but less likely to be reciprocal in giving you a chance to be able to do something you're passionate about.

One group I was with extended me the good fortune of educating me on just what patient-engaged research was all about, and they sent me for training in a Master Class on Patient Engaged Research. This group of people helped me a lot by really teaching me about this world, and offered me many unique opportunities to be part of their research into Primary Health Care. I learned a great deal from them, and they always treated me with respect. I remember telling them that a person comes to something like this not just because they want to help, but because there is always something they want too. I said I came to them because I had something that

I wanted, and that was to find some way to reach doctors and to get a chance to talk to them about addiction. Try as I may, I could not get into the University to speak to the medical students about addiction. They came up with all sorts of reasons why that could not happen. You'd swear I was trying to come in and contaminate them. It was only through the people on this committee that I was able to do this. They opened the door for me. I was very grateful for this.

I saw other places that gave patients the illusion that they were being offered the chance to contribute to decision-making, but really, they were being used to rubber stamp what they had already decided to do. In one incident the issue was restraint and seclusion policies, and the institution was telling the volunteer patient committee what to say regarding their feedback. They didn't bother to tell them why the issue had come up because it was related to a very public case that had been protested outside of the institution. They relied on the fact that the members would not know this and, being eager to please, would simply do as they asked. It was this kind of deceit that I found particularly disturbing. They were just using their patient partners.

I was asked by another doctor to become part of his research, and when I attended the first meeting, I discovered that what he wanted his patient partners to do was to take the secretary's notes, rent the room, and get the food for the meetings. I informed him that this was not the role of a patient partner, that he might want to inquire further into what the role was, and that taking their notes and renting the room, etc., was not something I was willing to do. This was another example of people just wanting to tick off a box because they were getting grants if they had patient partners. He hadn't even bothered to find out what role their patient partners should actually play in their research. Since I had taken a Master Class in Patient Oriented Research, I was very aware of what it was, so I was able to speak up, but had I not been there, that's what the other patient partners would have been doing.

I taught a session on being a patient partner at one institution to their volunteers. They had a speaker in the morning, and I was doing it in the afternoon. They paid the speaker in the morning, who was a person who did things in a volunteer capacity, $800.00 but refused to pay me because I volunteered at their institution.

I was asked to be on a committee to name a new program that was replacing an old one that had been operating there for some time, and there had been some community concerns expressed about this. The changes to the program had raised concerns for many people both inside and outside of the institution. The institution had replaced the addiction-trained staff with social workers, and there had been a lot of negative responses to this.

The whole exercise appeared to be a complete waste of time and some sort of deception, as nothing that we did during the meetings was ever used for anything related to the program. Once again it was the illusion of being asked to contribute, where there was absolutely no contribution ever really solicited or taken. It was as if they tried to create an act of deception to detract from the response they were getting initially. I described it as a game of smoke and mirrors.

In another invitation, many individuals from different agencies were invited by a large government-sponsored addiction agency to discuss the direction of substance abuse services. I was really impressed with their tactics. They determined where you were going to sit and with whom, what questions were going to be asked and answered, how they would be answered and how the output would be recorded. There was no way that you were going to have a chance to offer up anything other than what they wanted. I thought it was absolutely ingenious. They were able to control the people in the room so that, in the end, they could publish and have the perfect results that they initially wanted.

This agency would continue to prove over and over how it could control the narrative of substance abuse to the point where you could almost predict the direction that they were heading in just by watching what they were doing. You had to actually give a shit, though; otherwise, you just followed the person in front of you and hoped the funding came your way. In the end, it was always about getting the funding dollars and not about what was the most ethical thing you could be doing. These guys single-handedly changed the playing field so that addiction ceased to exist. They did this through their anti-stigma campaign, which hid the real agenda, which was to make addiction a choice and end the need for treatment. When addiction became substance use, and that became a choice, you no longer needed to treat it.

In one volunteer committee I was involved in, we could be involved with putting on a talk that was offered to the public, and I had offered to do one on addiction, since I had some knowledge of this subject. I used information from the American Surgeon General's Report that had just been released called, Facing Addiction in America. I wanted to present this and show how the neuroscience of addiction accurately predicted the lived experience and then introduce the ACE study. I was refused because I was told that they would not accept the research I chose because it had not been chosen by their clinicians, and the individual who spoke to me didn't agree with this research. This seemed ridiculous to me since the research was obviously sound given that it was the Surgeon General's Report.

At some point later, I ran into one of their clinicians who was sitting on a panel at a conference I was attending, that was supporting the exact same research. So, exactly what was this about? Why did they refuse the presentation? I gave this presentation later in Toronto and it was received very well, and I received many other requests to give the same presentation after this. I say this to show that the presentation was good, so why would they refuse it? It showed the neuroscience of addiction, which clearly supported the notion that addiction followed a neurological process that caused out-of-control use. The ACE study, which had been surfacing a lot around that time, was also speaking a lot about the fact that trauma had been the driving force behind addiction. The two general approaches that I was interested in were supported by the Alberta Family Initiative, which had put together The Brain Story, a nineteen-module course on how trauma affects the brain and how addiction and mental health are related to this, as well as numerous chronic illnesses and the importance of neuroscience in all of this.

This institution did do a presentation at the agency where I worked, which was an addiction agency, and they thought they should do a presentation on addiction, which was a mystery to me since we were an addiction agency, so I couldn't figure out what they thought we did. I had to assume that this was their standard presentation, and they never bothered to consider that maybe they needed to think through where they were presenting this. This could only be interpreted as laziness or arrogance because we sure as hell didn't need to be educated about addiction.

I once filled out a referral to them, but try as I may, I could not get it sent to them. I finally gave up and took a bus there and asked the receptionist to ask someone to come down from the unit and get the application. Later, when I called, I was told that they didn't take referrals. I asked them if this was true, why did they have an application on their website that said they did. I was told they didn't. I had to call the head of the unit, who then told me that there was an application online, and I suggested that they might want to inform their staff. I was then told that this wasn't how they did things, but they couldn't explain why their website clearly indicated that they did. This was the kind of insanity that you had to deal with. These were the state-of-the-art facilities that viewed you as not being educated enough to do the work, but they could not even figure out what they were doing.

When I did send clients over there they invariably did not end up where we were trying to get them referred to. If I sent them with a letter trying to explain what we were trying to refer them for and then accompanied them there, I was accused of trying to tell them what to do. I explained that I was simply trying to make sure what the program was, that we were trying to ask them to see if our client was suitable for, because every time we had sent them there, they kept sending them to another program we had not wanted them to go to. If they thought the person was unsuitable for that program, they simply needed to tell us that. These people very clearly didn't play well with others.

It was like waiting for the people who were supposed to do the Gain assessment for referral for treatment. That could take forever just to get the appointment for that, and then they'd choose a treatment center for your client. You'd look at their choice, and you'd know your client wouldn't last a day there. It was ridiculous. They didn't know your client worth a damn, and they obviously didn't know anything about the treatment centers either. There's no point in sending a client to a treatment center that gets in your face so that your client ends up kicked out the second day because he can't handle confrontation.

I was one person who, along with another, was responsible for bringing SMART recovery to our city. I could see that things were changing, and a lot of people had difficulties with twelve-step groups. I thought we could use some alternatives, and SMART recovery had looked like a good alternative. I ended up running a popular group out of the college where I used to work. I thought this would be a great opportunity for students taking the Addiction and Community Service Worker course to come in and learn to facilitate a group. I offered this to them. I said I would help them learn how to do it if they were interested. Interestingly, they didn't take advantage of this, but I ran the group anyway.

We had an Inuit treatment center that would bring their clients there, and this was amazing because I got to work with some of them in the group, and I ended up connected to many of them across the city as a result. It was a great honor for me. One problem emerged when one of the counselors who accompanied them and who sat in on the group violated the confidentiality rule of the group. She also worked part time in another agency. When one person who was a client of mine was accepted into that treatment center for long-term residential treatment, she revealed something she said in the self-help group, which resulted in getting the woman kicked out. This woman was trying to get as much treatment as possible because she had a very young child, and she wanted to be able to be the child's mother and to be able to be stable. Her mother, who had fourth-stage cancer, was taking care of her child until she finished this. She returned to the street after being kicked out and never came back to treatment.

I confronted the other counselor the following week and told her that the other woman was not welcomed back, and that she had no business repeating anything that was said by anyone at this meeting who was not from the treatment center they were with. I explained what had happened as a result and that this was unacceptable. I called the other treatment center, explaining that she had no business saying anything to them from a self-help group and that it was entirely out of context.

The director refused to acknowledge the inappropriate behavior of her employee and instead chose to accept it. This was clearly unethical but, as you can see, these places did not acknowledge ethics in their practices, and the results were extremely serious. I kept in touch with the client's mother, who managed to survive her cancer, but her daughter never did make it back to recovery and never became her daughter's mother. After such a clear violation of her confidentiality, would you blame this woman for never wanting to trust someone again?

There were treatment centers that were verbally abusive and used the clients to make money in a call center selling calendars. These were hyper-religious. There were treatment centers that still operated with the confrontation model and often publicly shamed people. Some of these places could do more harm than good, depending on who you sent there. Not all treatment centers were the same. Some treatment centers were OHIP covered, and others required that you pay for treatment. Some offered both, but the wait list for covered beds was long. You could send people out of the city if there weren't any services available in your own city. I could do a Gain assessment myself, so sometimes I would do the assessment myself if the treatment center would allow me to avoid the wait.

I sent one man over to a place where the receptionist thought that correcting the person's grammar was a good thing to do. Well, this guy had a mother who took great pleasure in doing that to him all the time and so he didn't react to her very well. All of a sudden, he had to leave because he wasn't acting appropriately. Well, go figure. This guy is unwell, which is why we're sending him there, and the little miss receptionist thought this was the day to correct his grammar without knowing anything about him. So now he doesn't get any help, but at least he got his grammar lesson for the day.

Where do they get their employees from? This was a concurrent disorders program. Could it not be assumed that the clients applying for services may not be functioning at their best when they come looking for services, so maybe their grammar isn't really the thing you need to focus on.

I've been working with a woman whose daughter has spent over twenty years on the streets using opiates, among other drugs. She's experienced every type of degradation and has had to live with an entirely different type of survival rules. Her mother says it's hard to see her or to spend time with her because her behavior and appearance is difficult to see, but she can't let her go, so she tries repeatably to help get her daughter into treatment. Sometimes she succeeds, but her daughter falls back to the streets, and a lot of times she just can't get things to line up because the expectations of the centers are too difficult for her daughter to manage to get in. She recently managed to make it work and she got her in, and it looked like it could work but her daughter stole a 79-cent bag of chocolate eggs from a gas station when she was out with the staff, and they kicked her out. They drove her to a shelter and drove off without checking to see if the shelter was full. This was all for a 79-cent bag of chocolate eggs. Her mother felt defeated. She said after all the work it took to get her in there, it was over just like that. She said the state of trauma was back, just like that. That constant state of fear of waiting for the call that says I'm sorry to tell you that your daughter is dead, all for the sake of a 79-cent bag of chocolate eggs. Life and death balanced on a 79-cent bag of chocolate eggs.

When I was working with kids, I referred a young girl to a youth psychiatry unit who had been affected by her mother's drug and alcohol use at birth. She was fifteen years old and the kind of kid who tried to help everyone else when no one was taking care of her. She had physical deformities at birth because of whatever her mother was consuming during the pregnancy. She was the kindest little girl. She had terrible organizational skills and just could not get it together if her life depended on it. She'd give you the shirt off of her back but often wasn't dressed warm enough in the winter. I was hoping that she could be evaluated and maybe get put on Ontario Disability Support Program (ODSP) so she could have a steady source of income. She would be plagued with issues for the rest of her life. Her family would never take care of her. If any kid deserved help, this kid did. I agreed to meet her before the appointment and accompany her because I knew how disorganized she was. She of course was late by about fifteen minutes, and I took her up to the youth unit.

When we got there, we were greeted by about four people, including the psychiatrist. The first thing she said was that if she couldn't even show up on time, why should they be bothered to help her? The little girl began to cry, which did not go well with me.

I looked at the psychiatrist and I said, "So, for the very reason that I referred her to you, you're telling her that you're not going to see her?" I continued: "I have already explained that I believe that she has been impacted at birth by her mother's drug and alcohol use, and you can see looking at her that she has facial deformities. She has serious organizational difficulties which affect her ability to get herself to places on time, like we have seen today, and this is what constitutes why you would not see her?"

The doctor began to quickly backtrack out of her original comment, but it is clear that if I had not been there my client would never have gotten any help.

You now must ask how many times that played out with other unaccompanied young people. What is wrong with this world where this woman has to start off so confrontational with a young girl so already harmed by the world she came into? This is what we can expect from the people who are supposed to be helping the most vulnerable members of our society. Is that really necessary?

We had another young man we sent over to a treatment program, and he came back worse than he was when we sent him. His drug use was completely out of control. The agency had not bothered to keep in touch with us or inform us of any problems they were having with him. We could have played a positive role in helping curb this situation if we had known what was happening, but this was another common tendency with other agencies. If they had your client, they refused to have any contact with you while they had them at their agency. This makes absolutely no sense whatsoever. After a while we had to stop sending our clients there because they kept coming back worse than when we sent them originally.

We required our clients to be abstinent because they were in a court-ordered program. We had a degree of leverage over them, and we could have contributed to helping our clients to stay on track while they were in their treatment centers. There was no reason why they could not have worked with us other than they simply refused to. The fact that this was going on and they had chosen not to tell us was a serious problem for both the client and our program.

Working with the Courts

I worked in a court program for a while, and that was another lesson in patience. In this case you were often taking clients from jail, which meant you usually had a housing issue and, most often, a methadone issue. This means you had to try and get these things set up so that when they were released you could take them to a pharmacy to get their methadone set up, and either have housing already arranged or have managed to convince detox to hold a bed for them. This would give you time to get them housing, but it would all have to be done after 2:00 pm when the court started and when they were brought to the court from the cells.

Essentially, this program offered people a chance to avoid jail if they did a treatment program and stopped using substances other than those prescribed. They came to the program every day, they got a very good food bank once a week, they had access to clothing, they were tested randomly, they had one-to-one counseling and group work, and they could have breakfast and lunch at the center every day.

If they did something wrong, they received sanctions like community service hours, and they would often argue about this, which, given all that they were given, often really surprised me. This amounts to volunteer hours and these guys would argue about this. They would argue if they tested positive, claiming they didn't use anything. This was a constant problem week after week.

They would often fight over the food bank, often hiding things from the others, until we had to lock the food bank up and then supervise them. You couldn't leave them in your office if you had to go and photocopy something for them because they stole from you. You had to tell them to leave your office and then lock it and go to the photocopy room. We had to let other employees know not to leave their office doors open or unlocked because they would steal from them. One of our clients walked out with one of the group room TVs. These were behaviors that they had engaged in prior to their arrest that were related to their addiction. This was part of what we were trying to address in treatment. We were treating both addiction and criminal behavior.

In court I had to sit back with them because their behavior was often inappropriate. They would either be lying down, playing with their phone or talking through the whole court session. It was also hard to get the judge to hold these clients accountable for their behaviors, which made working with them near impossible. One judge was more interested in being their friend than in dealing with the issues that were being raised. We were expected to go through all this work to make sure that they were where they said they were, which took up time we could be using for other more important things, and in the end, it was worthless, wasted time, because nothing would come of it. It was absolutely infuriating.

On one occasion, a worker was sitting in court with her client sleeping on her lap, who was snoring loudly. I couldn't believe it. I thought, "What the hell is this worker doing?" I was just so fed up that day that I texted my colleague and said I had to leave and then left the courtroom and went home. Some days it was just ridiculous. The person was quite capable of sitting on the bench. She's there because she's going to get a chance to avoid going to jail. She ran a rather lucrative drug dealing business. She could easily have managed to sit up. She wasn't incapable but she could get away with it. That's the point, she could get away with it. We treat addicted people like they are somehow unable to sit when, in fact, it just is not true. They are addicted and they cannot choose to stop. That is the truth. They can, however, sit.

This was just another example of how the system babies people with addiction. We acted like they couldn't manage. Here were people that were making thousands of dollars a week dealing drugs. They could buy their family members cars or a home, but they couldn't manage to sit up in a courtroom, and we were expected to buy into the fact that perhaps that's all they could do that day; they could just manage to show up and nap during the court process. It was an absolute joke. Some of these people had hurt people very seriously. Someone had cut people's fingers off. Someone used a hammer on people. They were capable of causing serious harm, but somehow, they couldn't sit.

In one instance, I was expected to go to the client's place to see if their residence was appropriate. I ended up in the most dangerous area in the city for drug dealing and crime. As we walked through the area, we were met by many people who knew the client, and she introduced me to them. Someone mentioned a shooting death that took place the day before. When we got to her place I was expected to look around for drugs or paraphernalia. She explained that she provided all sorts of things to her neighbors, including detergent and other necessities they might need. It was clear that everyone knew her and that she was most likely a dealer. She called her son down and introduced him to me and he was a huge man that towered over me. It was obvious that I wasn't safe in this area, and I was definitely not going to search this woman's place.

I went back to work and reported that we would have to accept this person as a client because I had just been identified by all the people in the neighborhood, so if this person did not gain entry into our program, I would be at risk. I also filed a safety report complaining that I didn't think that we should be doing these kinds of residential checks, given the obvious risks. So, we admitted a dealer into the program who was not addicted, and I ended up treating her for an addiction to power and money.

In our program, most of our clients were on methadone; if not they had to stop use on their own, and if they could not, then we sent them to detox. Some clients were sent to inpatient treatment if they continued to struggle. Some clients took off. We should have entitled our program the Games People Play because it really was all about the games. It was all about how to get one over on you. The biggest game was my urine may be positive for drugs, but I didn't use. So, it was how creative can you get with how you could have possibly gotten drugs into your system without having used. Now we had them sign a statement at the beginning saying that if they tested positive, they were positive, and how they were positive was not a subject for discussion, but that never seemed to matter. The ridiculous reasons continued to be given and to take up time in court, and they continued to gain some ground with these.

The reasons were creative. My girlfriend was using, and we had sex. I must have touched something that had some drug residue on it, and I wasn't aware of it. I was at a friend's place, and someone used. I left but I could have been contaminated. I was going through some of my stuff that I had left at my friend's, and I must have touched something. I had some things in storage and there might have been something on them. I walked by someone who was exhaling. I had some in my bra, but I didn't use it. Someone asked me to cut it, but I didn't use it.

The sanctions for these kinds of issues would be a recalibration of their clean time and community service hours. This would affect how long they would stay in the program with us and require that they volunteer somewhere in the community. I would see clients fight for extensive periods of time to lower the hours of community service, which at its most extreme might be ten hours, and most often five hours or less, to be completed in one week. They rarely spent a full day at the treatment center, so they had plenty of time to complete these.

These were people who were given a chance to avoid going to jail. They had usually committed a long list of crimes, and they had to complete a nine-month treatment program, and they were complaining about having to do volunteer hours. I found that absolutely insulting. It clearly showed their lack of appreciation for the opportunity that they had been given. That any judge entertained these arguments surprised me. Volunteering in the community is a prosocial activity and should be something we encourage in people who have been involved in antisocial behavior. Instead, it became an opportunity for clients to play games, at reducing their sanctions for violating the agreed-upon limitations on their behaviors while in the program. So, the very things we were trying to change in these clients were being reinforced by the courts.

It seemed to me that the courts wanted something to do, and so these ridiculous issues became things that they could argue about between the crown and the lawyers when, in truth, they were just a waste of time. They were also problematic for treatment because it placed the treatment team against the client.

The courts were clear on what we were expected to report on and how much we were supposed to keep track of, but whatever it was it was not of any great concern to the courts. If it was missing, we would be questioned about it for sure, but if it was there, it carried very little weight. The client could always find a way out of any issue that was raised. It appeared to be a lesson in futility and a huge waste of our time.

What I saw was that we taught people how to use the system to their own advantage. We taught them to be better users of the resources that were available. We taught them how to be more dishonest more effectively, and how to take more than what they needed. We taught them how to get away with more. This was common across all addiction services. The one thing we were really good at was teaching people how to use the system to get more than their share, to get more than they deserved, and how to do this repetitively.

One client I worked with ran a store out of her neighborhood. She not only sold drugs, but she sold lighters, cigarettes, meat, small bags of detergent, and just about anything else you could possibly need but not afford to buy. She would get larger quantities of things and then make small bags and sell those to her neighbors in a low-income neighborhood. I believe this happened with the food bank as well. They would take enormous amounts of food and then sell this to other people. All we ever succeeded in doing was creating a second economy for these people. We supplied the products that they could then sell for money to buy drugs. This is an insult to other people who have to rely on food banks and would never get the number of items that these clients received.

What we have done with people who are addicted, with all that we have handed out to them, is create very smart people who have become masters at taking from the system all that they can get. They know every loophole, every special circumstance, every place that gives out things and they make the rounds and get everything they can get. They'll fight each other to get the best stuff. When we had the food bank at work, people would sneak in and hide stuff that they wanted and didn't want to have to share with other members of the group before the time came to divide it up. They would get into fights with each other, and it wasn't because of scarcity because there was plenty of food. They wanted more. This is their economy, their free money. If you saw what they got, you would be shocked. Families in need do not get that much food.

I eventually left this program because I felt it missed the mark. I could not do the kind of work I wanted to do here. The chance to make meaningful changes in a person's life was limited by the program and the courts. There were too many different agendas running. The program was not cohesive. A court, by nature, is adversarial and it could not alter this to create something different in the case of a program that could bring about positive change. Its adversarial nature worked against this. A program that is at odds with itself leaves a weakness that the clients can exploit, and that's just what they did. They saw the weakness and they exploited it. It simply created a cat-and-mouse game that is not conducive to recovery from addiction.

This program should not have included Crown and Defense involvement in issues related to the clients' behaviors in the program and the issuing of sanctions and extension of their program. These were treatment issues and should never have been issues to be argued in court. The fact that they took away treatment's ability to have any meaningful effect on their client's ability to be successful in treatment. It made treatment ineffective. It made the court a joke, and it continually undermined the treatment counselors. The only time the court should have ruled is if the client absconded from the program, continued to use without the intention of stopping or showed no intention of complying with the program. The last two issues would have to be presented by the treatment team.

The reality is that the treatment team worked with the clients every day except weekends. They were able to see how the clients presented themselves in the center. They urine tested them. They checked their housing and did other follow-ups. They had the most contact with the clients, so they would be able to provide the most information. The clients were offered the program in order to avoid incarceration. This was the bonus they agreed to. This was their day in court.

They did not sign up to the treatment of their choice or to the idea that they could change the rules if they didn't like them. Working with people who have criminal backgrounds in a treatment program is hard work. Getting them to buy into the idea of treatment and changing their lives and their criminal ways of thinking is not easy. It is made much harder when you throw in a whole bunch of legal games, they can play with that are just not necessary.

When clients are trying to bargain to have one or two fewer hours of community service, when they have more than enough free time to do this, it is an insult to why we are giving them this chance in the first place. Community service is something people in recovery do as part of their recovery voluntarily. Why do we have to cajole these individuals who have violated the rights of everyday citizens through stealing and robbery into doing some volunteer work as a sanction? There is clearly something wrong with this program. How do we teach these people to become more prosocial if it is not through things like this?

The court was willing to give them the opportunity to find a way to avoid taking responsibility for their actions. They allowed them to challenge the treatment's assessment of them. These are the types of clients that are the most difficult to work with. Trying to challenge their criminal thinking and get them to change this to prosocial thinking is tough work. This was almost impossible when the courts gave them the opportunity to play games in the courtroom. It literally pitted the clients against the treatment team. It made further work at the treatment center almost impossible. They would come back so amused that they had got one over on treatment. It just created a toxic environment.

One of the things that I contributed to the program was that I drew a portrait of each of the clients that I gave them on the day of their graduation. I wanted to show them a picture of themselves minus the drugs they had been on when they entered the program nine months earlier. By then they usually looked much better than when they had arrived. They were often quite excited to see their portraits, and I really enjoyed doing this for them.

Working with Addicted Parents and Parents with Addicted Children

Another area that I found increasingly difficult in working in the addiction field was working with addicted parents. Having grown up in an addicted family, I knew only too well how damaging that can be. It was why I chose not to have children myself. I could not risk causing that sort of harm. Working with parents was extremely hard for me. I feared for their children. I knew the damage was already done, and I feared the damage they could still inflict. All of them laid claim to their children very adamantly, yet when they had been in their care they had been subjected to serious neglect and trauma. It was often their ownership that rang true. They are my kids, my child, and it was clear that they could do anything they wanted to them, or so they believed. This must be the darkest side of addiction.

I saw addicted people who used their kids because having kids allowed them to get more. Mothers who had babies because they wanted someone to love them. When the kid reached two, it was time to have another baby because this one had become too independent. They cast that kid to the side for the next baby. There were mothers too drugged out to know where their children were. There were those who left their children with strangers and didn't know what was happening to them. Children watching violence between their mother and whoever she brought home. Mothers who had one child after another, that they would eventually lose to CAS. Children who would be born addicted. I remember one doctor saying of those in jails and prisons that the majority had come from addicted homes.

The children who paid the penalty for being born. Blamed for their existence. Blamed for all the wrongs the mother experienced: "If it wasn't for you." "Look how much you cost me." "I never needed you." "What good are you?" How do you rise from that world? What sense of self can you actually have?

I read one of the most pivotal books once on child fatalities called Beyond Blame by Dr Peter Reder, Sylvia Duncan and Moira Gray. It was a study done in London, England. There was a comparable study done in Ontario. It described the conditions under which very young children end up losing their lives. In nearly all cases, the parents demand the children be returned to them if they have been taken from their care. Shortly after they're returned, they end up dead. The sense of ownership of the children is profound but it does not extend to the ability to care for the child. These are people who do not know how to love because they themselves have not been loved. They are looking for the child to love them.

There have been numerous cases of addicted parents tried for the murder of their very young children where addiction played a major role. Some of these have been covered in public trials. Two that come to mind are the Groves trial, where both parents were using methamphetamine and, after the mother caused the death of their very young infant son by beating him, they both participated in hiding his body by burying him in two milk crates and then weighing them down and dumping them into a deep well on their property. The other case concerns a mother, Jhenea Pratt, who gave her eighteen-month-old daughter a sippy cup with fentanyl in it so she could relax and smoke pot without the baby bothering her.

I had my own experience with an alcoholic mother, and that did not go well for me. I had been completely robbed of my childhood and left to believe that I was the mistake that should never have been born. The experience I had as a child impacted my entire life. When the person who gave birth to you constantly undermines your sense of self and can do this for all your formative years, unraveling that later on is very difficult. The fact that my mother predicted her death on my nineteenth birthday and then died a day and a month before I turned nineteen gave me no way to sort this out with her. The fact that I loved her deeply left me in a state of deep confusion for a long time.

Then there are the parents of addicted kids, and they can be children of all ages. These are the family members they are not allowed to grieve for. No one wants to hear about it. "Just forget about them." "Just walk away, after all look at them, they deserve whatever happens to them." "Didn't they steal from you?" "Didn't your son wreck your car?" "Didn't your daughter steal forty dollars from your wallet?" "Why do you bother worrying about them? I'm sure they're not thinking a damn about you."

So, they suffer in silence, fearing that they might get the call that their child might be found dead. They find out that their daughter's been beaten up badly by some guy she was staying with. They go to meet her to see if they can find her somewhere to stay. It's horrible. Her face is a mess. None of the shelters want to take her. She's broken the rules at one place and the others are too full. You can't take her home because she wrecked the place the last time. You pay for a few nights in a rooming house and go home. You promised you weren't going to do that again, but you can't just walk away. Nobody cares. Everyone says they have enough services but it's a lie. There aren't any. You've been to enough places with her and gotten that look of despise enough times to know they see you the same way they see your child. Could you please take the trash out with you?

At home you can't talk about it because no one wants to hear about it. Your friend talks about how well their daughter is doing in their new job and how she is looking forward to a holiday abroad with her fiancé. There's definitely a wedding in the works soon. She says her son is finishing his BA and will be doing a master's in science. You have nothing to say because there isn't anything to say. You feel the pain in your heart for the child you wish you could watch get married or graduate. All you can hope for is that maybe they'll live another day. It's the secret sadness you can't talk about. It's the secret fear that just sits there somewhere in your chest, and when you're driving home, you're afraid to see her on a street corner. You can only truly get this if you're one of these people. I have listened to enough of these parents to know the level of pain they live with. They are the people somehow unentitled to their grief. One Harm Reduction advocate told one parent about her thirty-eight-year-old daughter that she could live another decade on the street as if this was in any way good news.

What Was Going On in the Addiction Field?

I attended a conference put on by a major Canadian Center focused on Substance Abuse, where I was presenting a poster on Lived Experience of Addiction and Neuroscience and the Ace Study. I had tried to enter it as a presentation, but it wasn't accepted. While there, I attended a talk given by the People Who Use Drugs, who I had not heard of before. I was very curious about this group, which was why I attended. I was in for a shock. This presentation focused on what this group wanted to be given when asked to present at any conferences as experts on people who use drugs.

They requested that they be given a room where they could use their drugs and that there be no medical personnel present in that room. They wanted some of the newer paraphernalia available to them. That would be cookers for heating up their opiates. They wanted to be paid in cash and not in gift cards. They wanted their travel costs and hotel accommodation paid for. They wanted someone to have checked out ahead of time where they could procure their drugs if this was a different city. They did not want pro-recovery people anywhere near the room where they would be consuming their drugs.

Two of the lead people who were part of this organization had died. Now, just in case you don't get the significance of these requests, let me break it down for you. Wanting cash is just better for paying the dealers, they prefer it. Of course, they don't want to have to go looking for their drugs, so it would be handy if you take care of that. Can you imagine what a buzz kill it would be to have those do-gooder recovery people around when you're trying to get high? And it's no surprise that two of their organization members had died since this lifestyle choice isn't the healthiest. I'd like to say that I've spoken at these events, and they never paid for my accommodation or travel.

When I heard this person's presentation, I was shocked. I couldn't believe that I was hearing this at this conference. I felt like it was some sort of joke or mistake. I thought we couldn't have possibly come to this. We couldn't have possibly reached a point where we thought that this was in any way acceptable. She had mentioned something about her concern about someone having had CAS involved in her life and how unfair this was. I had commented at the end about the effect of drug use on children, and she had commented back that alcoholism affected children as if opiates did not. Interestingly, there was a recent news release about a couple that injected their three children under the age of six with heroin in order to keep them quiet while they used it. Her notion that people using opiates somehow made better parents was just ridiculous. And therein lies the problem. When people suffer from addiction, they are not capable of rational thought. It was easy to detect that she was under the influence during the presentation. It was also obvious that someone else had produced the slides for the presentation, which were acknowledged in the presentation.

I created a video that addressed my views on this presentation and posted it to YouTube. I started posting videos on my feelings regarding addiction because I felt I was in a unique situation to be able to offer some honest views on the subject. I had firsthand experience, and I wanted to give people some emotional accounts of firsthand experiences. After attending the Conference, I wanted to comment on how I felt about this particular presentation. A while after I had posted it, I discovered it had been removed, and the reason cited was that the person who posted it had closed their account. Well, I was the poster, and I had not closed my account, so I posted it again. It certainly made me curious about why it had been removed.

So why was this effort being made to support this presentation? What was behind this? My belief is this: it is what is being supported as the new less costly drug policy. Support drug use. It's less costly than treating addiction. We no longer have an addiction problem; we have a drug use problem. We just need to help people get their use sorted out. We teach people how to use it in a non-problematic way, and that's the answer. Give people twelve sessions of counseling. That's all they need. We don't need to do more than that. Let people decide what they want to do. People using drugs is less costly than helping people to stop using drugs. We currently prescribe all these drugs for people who are addicted, therefore there is no problem. It was a sobering thought.

I had left the last agency I was at, working full time as an addiction counselor. I had grown tired of working in an unhealthy work environment. For the majority of my time working in this field I never made more than $19.00 an hour. We had brought a union in there, and we managed to up our wages to about $26.00 an hour. I had managed to become a Registered Psychotherapist. It was something the agency encouraged, but it did nothing to improve our pay.

There were many things about that agency that made me question the work I was doing. Events took place that I reported to my manager that I felt should have been followed up on that never were. I have already mentioned those, and they were the type of things that stay with you. You can only accumulate so many of these kinds of things before they take a serious toll on you.

There were also incidents with staff that were very difficult, and that became serious enough that continuing to work there became dangerous to my mental health, and so I chose to leave.

I realized that the field was changing in ways that were making working in it something I wasn't sure if I could continue to do in good faith. I decided to take a part time job in an agency that I had known for many years and that had a great history in the community as always being very recovery oriented. It was founded by a wonderful woman who was a real pillar in the recovery community. She had passed away very recently, but her memory was not going to. I thought that here I could still do some work and that it would be the type of work that I really wanted to do.

I took the position, and I was clearly told that I would be working with people in recovery and not with people who were still actively using. I made a point to say that I had enough of that type of work and really was looking forward to working with people in recovery. It was clear from the beginning that the staff and the director were not as familiar with addiction, and we began seeing some very sick people showing up and people who were very addicted and also parenting young children. I made a point to say that I didn't think that we were the right agency to be working with this type of client, especially when there were young children involved because we were outpatient. We couldn't monitor the situation close enough to ensure the children were safe.

There were some very serious situations that occurred. I asked again why we were working with these clients, given the seriousness of their situation. I asked why I had been told that we weren't going to be dealing with this, and now we were. This was exactly the reason I no longer wanted to work with actively using people because when children were involved, you often had to deal with serious trauma incidents to the children, and I had dealt with far too much of that sort of thing previously. You end up with Secondary Traumatic Stress.

One of the clients they referred to me was involved with an infant whose injuries were horrific. It seemed like the director did not understand that addiction and young children did not make for a safe situation. In this case the drug was methamphetamine. I sent a research article to the director and the staff detailing the danger of having parents who are using this drug caring for young children. It seemed like they still didn't get it. It wasn't until I attended a board meeting where I brought up my concerns that I was finally heard.

This was exactly what I was trying to get away from. What resulted from my expressing my concerns was that I was asked, along with another employee, to conduct client screenings. We were to screen the clients in order to screen out those who were not appropriate for the agency.

Despite this I continued to see clients that were using and had young children. They only sent some clients for referrals for screening. The family who I had mentioned was still being seen by the agency, and I asked again why this family was still seeking services with us when it was more than obvious, we were in no way able to deal with the seriousness of their case. They wanted the return of their baby when the injuries to that child had been of such severity that you needed to be very careful how you proceeded. These parents should have been sent to residential treatment to ensure they had no chance of harming their child again. It was clear that this agency lacked the knowledge of addiction to deal with these sorts of extreme cases.

There was a decision to hire a consultant who was a person that I personally knew. This person was a pro-harm reduction person. Three weeks after she was hired, my contract was terminated because I was told that they didn't share my philosophies. There had been a discussion on harm reduction the week before, and I had said that I didn't see why we needed to go that route since many other agencies already practiced harm reduction.

I said that traditionally this agency had been abstinence-based, and I didn't see the need for this to change. The conference organizers were having another presentation with the same presenter from the People Who Use Drugs, and I said that this was an example of where that philosophy was going, and I felt that this was as far from recovery as you could possibly get. I suggested that she might want to check it out. This was the conversation that ended my employment.

This was the point where I realized that I no longer belonged in this area of employment at all. When I looked back over my history of involvement with Addiction and Mental Health, I couldn't see much of anything I could say that was positive or truly helpful. I saw a lot of half-hearted attempts to appear like we were trying to help people, and that is not to say that some people weren't helped. Despite the limitations that were constantly leveled against this area of intervention some people did manage to get well. If you really cared, it was painful. Sometimes, despite the agencies you worked for, you could continue to try and help someone, even when the agency told you to just give up, and that would make a difference for them, and they would make it.

There were times when it was a constant fight with every other agency that you had to engage with. There were the hospitals that didn't want to have anything to do with your clients because they just didn't see them as worth helping. There were mental health facilities that just wouldn't see your clients and would give you no explanation as to why. If you tried to advocate on their behalf, they accused you of trying to tell them what to do. Instead of collaboration you encountered the attitude of an adversary. Meanwhile, real lives hung in the balance. At times it felt like you were fighting a constant battle to try and get your client the help they needed. There were so many obstacles to overcome, the chances were slim that you would ever succeed.

The degree of dysfunctional people who worked inside the agencies that worked for addiction and mental health was also surprising. That was also something I saw firsthand throughout the time that I worked in this field. From misleading the public to taking advantage of volunteer groups, agencies didn't seem to think that they needed to, or would ever be held accountable for, their improper behaviors and the sad reality was they rarely were. It was sad to see that people could die as a direct result of the incompetence of the people and institutions that were working with them, and they would never get any justice for their deaths. It seems that having a diagnosis of addiction meant you could be mistreated and die without any repercussions.

I wish we could use another name other than harm reduction because that's just not what it is. They hide behind that idea as if that is what they are talking about, but it isn't. That's how they make anyone who opposes them look bad. I don't oppose harm reduction. I oppose no recovery whatsoever. I believe in methadone for opiate users. I believe in needle exchange, injection sites, Narcan, and clean supplies. What I don't believe in is giving up and supporting addiction. I don't believe in giving addicted people all of the drugs they want. I do believe in trying to encourage them to try and stop their addiction. I do believe in treatment for addiction. Look at Kensington Ave in Philadelphia. Is that what we really want? It looks like the zombie apocalypse. Do we consider that a humanitarian effort? I think the more appropriate name for what is currently happening is not Harm Reduction but Sustaining Addiction. We are currently applying the Sustaining Addiction Approach.

I had clients on the full cocktail of methadone, benzodiazepines, and amphetamines, along with other psychiatric drugs. This was considered "Your Recovery, Your Way." One young man continuously became psychotic from the amphetamines, and we would try and get him admitted until the amphetamines wore off so he would become non-psychotic, but the doctors wouldn't keep him. We tried to get the doctor and pharmacy to stop dispensing the amphetamines, but they refused to do this. His behavior was quite bizarre because he believed a microchip had been planted in his brain and he was being watched so he was considering going into the wilderness until the batteries ran out. Unfortunately, it was winter, and we were concerned he could freeze to death if he did this. These kinds of problems were just not considered and not responded to. As long as the client wanted the drugs, he got them regardless of whether they were causing any harm.

The Sun ran an article on August 12, 2022, concerning a local real estate owner who was asking the city to buy his apartment building because he could not rent his apartments. He said its nearness to a consumption site for drug use made them unrentable because his front lawn was forever covered in dirty needles despite the needle disposal boxes. The reality is that people who are using drugs are unlikely to be conscientious about where they discard their used needles. The other problem was keeping these people from breaking into the apartments. I can share some of these difficulties because I live in Vanier, where one of the neighbors in the apartment where I live has reported being very disturbed when a woman brought a client to our laneway to have oral sex right outside her daughter's bedroom window. I'm sure for those lucky enough not to have to live in these areas this must not even have to occur to them. So, I'm sure Harm Reduction is working for some, but for others it's not.

We have this distorted idea that all we have to do is provide drugs for addicted people, and all will be well. We somehow assume that when people are under the influence of drugs and alcohol, they behave well. I have no idea where anyone got this idea from or whether it is simply that they are banking on the fact that these people will not be in their neighborhoods, so it won't matter to them. Intoxicated people are unable to be considerate of other people because they are intoxicated, and this state of mind doesn't allow them to take others into consideration. They are unlikely to clean up after themselves because they are not able to focus on such things while intoxicated. Anyone who has worked closely with addicted people can give you plenty of stories about what happens around intoxicated people. Check out the shelters or John Howard Housing to e how absolutely frightening things can get. Getting their drugs is not their only problem.

We developed a problem in my neighborhood. Actually, it's the apartment building where I live. I live beside a house that, for the entire time I have lived there, has been inhabited by people who are actively using drugs. There used to be a wall that separated their backyard from our laneway, but it was broken down last year. Since then, they have begun to threaten one of my neighbors who parks her car there. They were sending their dog over to our back area to do his business, and when she asked them to stop doing this, they began a reign of terror over her. They slashed her tires three times, they keyed her car, and they finally smashed her windshield.

They see our laneway as theirs now. It gives them and their friends access to their backyard from the street. She has installed cameras because, without absolute proof, she can't do anything about what they've done. They threatened her and called her names every time she came home from work. This is a real problem with people who are using drugs because they do not behave in ways that make living near them an easy thing. They will intrude into your life without thinking and threaten you if you object.

There is another house that is behind me on another street where I routinely am bombarded by this man's rant about his girlfriend as he pounds on the door, demanding his belongings be returned to him. This happens at any time of night and day, and it can go on for up to an hour at a time. This gets mixed in with the gunshots and the sirens. I am at a loss as to where anyone gets the idea that people using drugs do not cause problems for others.

I often look at the United States because they are usually ahead of us in what they are doing about addiction. I think they have gone the way of harm reduction and open-air drug use, and they are beginning to see how that has played out, with Kensington Avenue being a good example of how this just has not worked. They have blocks upon blocks of people who look half dead amongst the never-ending piles of rubbish. People are tired of it. It's a nasty scene.

There's a YouTube channel where a guy just drives around and around it every day. If they didn't tell you what it was, you might think you were watching "The Walking Dead." The current drug-using trend is Fentanyl plus an animal tranquilizer called Xylazine, so the people are frozen in a bent-over pose for very long periods. They look like they just bent over to tie their shoes and froze there.

They are now realizing that this might not have been the best idea and are reconsidering the idea of abstinence. And here's the problem that I get tired of. I've been watching this problem now for over twenty years, and I've seen varying responses. I've watched the pendulum swing back and forth. Sometimes I think our responses have been as little thought out as if they were just blown in with the wind.

There has often been a big focus on language, as if that is all we really need to do. If we come up with the right language everything will suddenly change. For me the focus on language has been like the magician's sleight of hand. "Watch the ball, I'm going to put it under one of these cups, and then I'm going to move the cups around. Keep your eye on the cup with the ball under it. Now, see if you can figure out where the ball is." Really the ball is gone. It was never in play. It was never under the cup in the first place. Fooled you.

I think everyone knows it's not our agenda. It's not the agenda of the people on the right side of the issue. It's not for the greater good. There's a whole lot of other things at play here, and we need to get honest about that but who really wants to get honest about that? Addiction is a tricky subject. It comes with a whole lot of issues that are subjects we'd rather not put on the table. It was a lot easier when we could just view these people as the cause of their own problems and leave it at that, but the long and winding road to the present has made things much messier.

Today, addicted people occupy this strange space where we see them as unable to do anything with any intent whatsoever. They are seen in this helpless way and so we must just coddle them and accept whatever behavior they display because they are unable to do anything else. I was told that at one injection site, a person came in and just defecated on the floor. One employee brought this to the attention of the manager, who simply said this was OK; they probably couldn't do much better. I am amazed and shocked by the absolute insanity of people working in these places. I have to ask who is more ill, the addicted person or the people working at these facilities. They do this because they know you are stupid enough to accept whatever they do. You are encouraging these behaviors and turning these people into animals. What the hell is wrong with you? Have you lost your mind? The next thing you'll be doing is diapering them. Where do you get the people who work in these places? They can't possibly have any education in addiction. I think we should check to see if they have suffered some sort of brain damage because the ideas that they are buying into are just ridiculous. If they are true, then these people need to be hospitalized because they have reached the point where they can't care for themselves. It's either one or the other but both can't be true.

Let's do a Recap on the History

We started with those weak-willed people who just could not control themselves and had to keep using substances until they made a nuisance of themselves. They couldn't drink or use substances like other people. No, they had to go overboard and act like complete fools and become a problem. Over the years they got worse and became thieves and robbers and had to be arrested and jailed as the substances of abuse became more serious. They could be violent and dangerous, and they could destroy property, and they could never be trusted.

This then became the people who had a medical disease and needed treatment for it. They were sick and couldn't help themselves and needed to be helped to get better. This began the AA movement and subsequent twelve-step movements and treatment centers that employed the confrontational tear you down and build you up approaches because, after all, they still saw you as morally bankrupt. You needed to be forced back into shape.

Eventually this seemed a bit extreme, and there was a movement to see addicted people a bit more compassionately. This began the idea that if you changed the language, the attitudes would change. Stop calling people addicts and suddenly everyone would see them differently. There was a grassroots movement that involved the recovery movement, and this included the film "The Anonymous People" and people like Bill White.

It looked like the recovery movement was about to lead a revolution of change. We would now be people in long-term recovery. In the US, they would have recovering community centers, recovery high schools and colleges and people would march on the street for recovery.

In Canada, we had the Faces and Voices of Recovery, which began in Vancouver. They tried to set off the same movement here. In Ottawa, we had a recovery peer group, which began to have Recovery Day, a one-day event to celebrate recovery from addiction. There was some conflict with the twelve-step movement, which did not believe in being in the public eye, and they didn't like the change from identifying as an alcoholic or an addict to a person in recovery.

Recovery Day was asking people to come down and celebrate their recovery at City Hall where everyone could see them. The twelve-step program's traditions stated that we needed to remain anonymous at the level of press, radio and films. This event would attract the press, so it conflicted with the very people it was trying to celebrate, and if you think the addiction agencies had a hard time getting along with each other, this was not an easy alliance either.

The twelve-steps have a tradition that asks us to place principles before personalities, and this is not without reason. There are a lot of very big personalities in the twelve-step programs. You can often see this in their business meetings or any of their committee meetings. Strong personalities emerge, and the meetings can often be rather high-spirited and filled with hot debate. They created the twelve traditions to help with this and they take these rather seriously, hence why they had difficulty with the idea of making any public appearances. It took a while to get the recovering community to feel comfortable enough to come out.

Some of what this group of people were trying to do was to change the language that recovering people were using to refer to themselves, and they offered some training to help people grasp these ideas. This was done through info from Voices and Faces of Recovery and through showing the film "The Anonymous People." They were teaching people to see themselves differently and to speak about themselves differently.

The film "The Anonymous People" was an almost contagious message of a movement that started in the United States. As it followed the movement, you saw into the lives of ordinary people and some famous people who played a part in this movement. You saw people graduating from high schools and universities that had supported their recovery. You saw people walking into community centers that were run *by* recovering people *for* recovering people. You saw members of political parties who were part of the recovering community. You saw masses of recovering people marching in the streets wearing colorful t-shirts announcing their recovery group. By the time the film ended, you were ready to say sign me up. It was such a positive message, and I don't think people had seen such a positive recovery message before and I think it was long overdue.

Those who were organizing Recovery Day also reached out to the Addiction Agencies and anyone else who had a part to play in the treatment or the education of addiction. It set out to play a pivotal part in the world of addiction treatment and the lives of recovering people. The people who gathered around that idea had dreams that paralleled what they saw in the film "The Anonymous People." They dreamed of a city that had a place for recovery where recovering people could go. They dreamed of a city that celebrated recovery. They dreamed of a time when prejudices would be gone.

Unfortunately, not everyone who came to the table shared the same dream, and there were others who had their own ideas of where they thought the world of addiction should go. There would be those who would take advantage of the ideas that were part of this dream. They would use them for their own ends. The recovering people themselves were vulnerable. They did not all have the expertise to compete with the professional people they attracted to their cause. They ran the risk of being co-opted into someone else's agenda, and they were.

One problem that emerged in Ottawa was the rise of a local peer group and the attention of the government agency for substance use. The peer group created a Recovery Day event and opened this up for addiction agencies to be present. There was one individual who put himself forward as the face of recovery day. He put himself strategically in the center of that event. He then went on a circuit promoting himself as the face of recovery. This gave him the ability to travel and create a portfolio of himself in various cities around the world, forever holding the Recovery Day Ottawa sign with all sorts of people, including some who were well known. This also placed him strategically in the right place to be the main communicator between the recovering community and the professional organizations.

Did he have the necessary prerequisites for this? No, he did not. He had worked in a low-level job in a treatment center and had taken some education in addiction. I don't believe he was able to have a critical appraisal of the people who invited him into their circles and, to be fair, these people would be the people who would be able to offer this peer group the difference between successful financial survival and a continual low-level struggle. Despite the ideas held by the peer group, they would be influenced by the government agency if they were to survive financially. So, although recovery was initially the prime focus of this peer group, this would be altered with this association.

This is where the linguistic sleight of hand showed up. The Government agency involved in substance use joined the strategy to change the language around addiction as a way to reduce stigma. The recovery people had viewed this as identifying as *people in recovery* rather than as identifying as an addict or an alcoholic, which had been the case up to that point among people in recovery.

The government agency determined that addiction was not a positive word, so it should be done away with, and the language should be changed to a substance use disorder, or a person should be referred to as *someone who uses substances.* The removal of the word addiction neatly removed the idea that a person was addicted. They avoided the idea of recovery because if they removed the idea of addiction there would be no need for recovery.

People were now just using substances. They might have some issues with their use, but they would never be addicted. If there was no such thing as addiction, there was no need to treat it, and if people were simply choosing to use substances, then that was their right, and no one had a right to suggest that they shouldn't use them. The change in language had quite an impact on how we looked at what once was a problem. The problem with this is addiction continues to exist. Nothing has changed but the language.

This was a substantial departure from the goals or aims of the recovering community. They had not sought to legitimize using drugs and alcohol but to celebrate recovery. They believed that people became addicted and that they could recover from addiction, and they wanted to celebrate this. They had no idea what the government was up to nor that they had been co-opted into this much broader view of substance use that now included people who used substances and should be supported for using substances.

The most recent effect of the marriage of this Government Agency involved in substance use and the Ottawa peer organization of recovering people showed up in the disappearance of Recovery Day since 2022 and its replacement with the WOW Festival. One of the first things to emerge out of the formation of Ottawa's first addiction peer group was its Recovery Day event. This brought recovering people together to celebrate their recovery from addiction. This was following what was seen in "The Anonymous People" video. This has changed, but not surprisingly when you look at the financial disclosure for Ottawa's addiction peer group, which reveals that $460,000.00 of its revenue is coming from government funding. Government funding has always controlled the direction of the addiction treatment world, so why shouldn't it control the peer support world as well? So, if there is no need for recovery, we do not need Recovery Day.

I spoke to the gentleman who became the spokesperson for Recovery Day, and he had learned the message. He needed to go with the change. The new understanding was that we should be trying to support the people who had a right to use substances if that was something they preferred. There had to be a space for all the people. In that moment I thought perhaps he had drunk the Kool-Aid too. We know that these are not people who are social users. These are people who have problematic use. It was like saying we should support active addiction as well because, after all, some people just like it that way. I had a hard time trying to figure out how he made sense of that.

So Where Does All This Leave Us?

There has been a serious change that has seemingly gone unnoticed. Harm reduction has now taken on a new and very different meaning. Harm reduction now means sustaining addiction at any cost. For all those related to someone with serious substance abuse disorder, they must accept that their loved one lives a hellish life in a dark and ugly world. There is no way to retrieve them from that world. They may come back to them when they are beaten and broke, looking for money or something else they want them to give them before returning to that world. The Harm Reductionists will tell them not to worry because they can live a long time like that, as if that is some sort of relief and not a worse horror. They will pat themselves on the back for the great work they are doing and be grateful they got rid of the likes of me.

It's like the world they create is not the nightmare that it is. I come back to the reality that they often don't live in their neighborhoods. They don't see the fallout of their idea of the right way to treat substance abuse. They don't hear the gunshots at three in the morning or watch the faces of the people who are no longer there, stumbling down the streets of their neighborhood. It's the faces of hopelessness and despair. There isn't anyone behind their eyes. The lights have gone out. They are enslaved to addiction. They have no choice, and only somebody who has been there knows that reality. I lived in that reality. For the longest time death looked like the only way out. Carelessness was the way I flirted with death. I played with the drugs, hoping I would accidentally cross the line and not come back. The desire for death became my closest companion. I sought out treatment because death would not come quickly enough.

Let's look at some of the most negative consequences of being addicted. I'd like to start with a pamphlet I walked by in my neighborhood for many years and one I often stopped and looked at, wondering to myself if this woman was ever going to be found. Her name was Mary. She was Inuit, and she disappeared five years ago. She was found in Oct 2022 on Deschamps Street when they were doing some construction on an apartment building.

There had been other women in Vanier that had died because they had been addicted, because these are women that are often targeted because no one will notice, or when they are reported missing, no one will take that seriously.

Vancouver's downtown eastside has seen one of the most disturbing examples of this. Willie Pickton had taken the lives of many more women than he would ever be charged with. His crimes would go unnoticed for so long because addiction somehow made these women's lives lack any value at all. Each of those women had a story that explained why they had ended up on the downtown East Side, and each story was heartbreaking. I know because I took the time to read about them. To be left as if your life has no meaning in this world is a crime. It was why I could not just walk by that pamphlet in my neighborhood without thinking about Mary every time and wondering where she was and when she would be found.

How dare any of us presume to think it doesn't matter because this person was addicted? This was someone's sister, someone's mother, someone's daughter and a person who was loved by her people. We don't get to disregard that, ever.

Just recently I watched the news reported that police were forcibly removing the homeless off the streets of Vancouver's downtown East Side, which is home to many addicted people, while BC Housing announced clearly that they had no housing to offer these people.

I kept wondering what the aim of all this was. Where was this heading?

During the period of the reported evictions this poster was found posted:

> *Attention Homeless:*
> *Tents and belongings on the sidewalks will be burned with gasoline and propane canisters.*
> *Residents that live in the area, we will not allow you to destroy our community any longer with your selfishness.*
> *You have seven days to comply.*
> *This is a serious warning to the homeless in the area.*
> *Leave now or suffer the consequences of your selfish addiction!*
> *Insite: the safe injection site will be the first building to be burned down if the homeless and addicted humans do not leave the area in the seven-day period.*
> *Last and final promise.*

Around this same time, a stranger doused a woman with gasoline and set her on fire, and a man's belongings were set on fire.

It was clear hatred was building. If you walked the Downtown East Side of Vancouver, what you saw was blocks of streets that had become lined with tents. There had been storefronts there at one time and there were still some businesses attempting to operate. For the most part, all building entrances were blocked by the tents and makeshift shelters that the homeless had erected. Some of the homeless had items laid out on blankets that they were selling. I had been in the area twice and walked through it, and it was frightening. People injected themselves in full view. People dressed outside in full view. The second time I was there it had become much more dangerous. You clearly sensed you were not welcome.

Addiction is not an easy subject to discuss, but if you're going to discuss it you need to be completely honest about it. You can't paint a picture that only gives a partial story, so you get what you want by telling it that way. For God's sake let's just be honest and tell the whole story and be done with it. Believe me, if we hear the whole story, we should clearly want to do something about it because it's a bloody horror story. All we get with our partial truths is responses that do nothing for one group while helping another, and the problems just continue to fester.

Addiction has a profound effect on a huge number of people and not just on those who are addicted. Painting the addicted as nothing but victims and denying that they impact innocent others is infuriating to the people they impact. These people are also victims of addiction. In our current climate, the government thinks that if it just claims that addiction no longer exists, it will have solved the problem, meanwhile cashing in on the proceeds of it.

With the government organization, The Canadian Center for Substance Use, supporting the Association of People Who Use Drugs, what message are they sending?

The sad thing about addiction is what caused it in the first place. It was the fact that the person was wounded before they became addicted, and that's why they were at risk of addiction. It's like the insult of the whole thing. Unprotected children are left at risk and then wounded as children. Not enough protection for children and the tendency to protect parental rights no matter what. No recognition that children need help for what has happened to them, and there are not enough resources available to even give them help if it was recognized they needed it. It's the recipe for addiction, and it's not fair.

It's the constant failure of our system that supplies the

endless numbers of future addicted people, and then we dare to say, well, they should have the right to use, which is, in my opinion, the ultimate betrayal. It is the absolute minimum we are prepared to do, and it is lining somebody's pockets. Everybody's cashing in on the misery of these people, and the Harm Reductionists are just as much a part of that system as those who are benefiting from the sale of the drugs. They have systematically moved in to take over the treatment system. They have been able to get rid of every person who holds a different opinion than theirs because they are endorsed by the funders. It is only a matter of time before they are the only position that exists.

The biggest funder of addiction treatment is the government, and the government has more to gain by supporting people's right to use than it does by supporting abstinence. The largest consumers of legal addictive items are those who have a problem. They consume the largest amount and therefore provide the largest profit. We are talking about numbers in the area of billions of dollars. This is not something to take lightly. Our government makes considerable money from the sale of alcohol, tobacco, pot, gambling, and lottery. It's a lot cheaper to support the idea of people's right to use than sending them to treatment for addiction. If people continue to use, the government continues to make money and save money.

It's time people saw this for what it is. We can go on being ignorant of what is actually taking place, or we can open our eyes and see things for what they are. Let's be realistic. There are no really nice guys out there. I foolishly thought that when I first stepped into the field. I was full of all the bright notions of doing the right thing. Over and over, what I actually found was one after another of self-centered, greedy, power-hungry people who, for the most part, only cared about themselves.

I was wide-eyed and a little too green. I thought people really cared. I no longer think that anymore. What I ran into over and over I can barely understand. It boggles my mind. Who out there ever acted in good faith for the good of the people they were claiming to help? They were far and few to find. Most people were looking for power and control. Most people were focused on themselves. The person they were helping seemed to be an afterthought. In the end it seemed to be all about them.

The conclusion I have come to as to where all of this is going to is when I realized that in March of 2024, the MAID law would be open to people with Mental Health Issues and of course that would include people with addiction. It was then that I could see why letting the addicted use made sense. You see, if you've been addicted, you know that the drugs don't really work after a while, and you end up just having to use because you are addicted and not because they do anything for you anymore. That was the trap that I found myself in at the end of my use. Well now you can choose suicide, and the government will help you with that. So, they'll assist you to keep using until that dead end becomes the dead end that it is, and death becomes the only way out. Then they'll kindly help you with that. I have heard that they have chosen to delay this decision, but it will get there. That's what they want, an easy way to rid them of the problem.

This has been one of the most difficult journeys of my life. I think it was so difficult because so much of my life had been tied up in it. To be born into the world of addiction and to have had my family so damaged by it, and my own life so destroyed by it as a child, was huge for me. The consequences would shape my life, and the trauma so impacted me that it would follow me throughout my adult years. I would never have a normal life. It would cost me that. I would never have children, and I would never have a loving relationship. I lost that to that trauma. In the end I would live my life alone. There would often be a great sadness that would follow me.

My friends would say I was loved, but they did not spend the endless time I spent alone. I helped many people, and I fought for the rights of many people, and I am glad that I did that. I am proud of the work that I did.

I carried a lot of traumas from my adult life, as well as from my own years of addiction. I suffered years of trying to get well from a mental health condition. When I clearly saw all the damage that addiction could cause in my life and the lives of others, I was moved to want to do something about that. I believed that I could do something. I believed that I was intelligent enough that I could make a meaningful contribution. I thought that this would be a noble thing to dedicate my life to. This would be something meaningful. I never dreamt that I would enter into a world that would so oppose the idea of actually helping. I hadn't prepared myself for the amount of shocking distastefulness I would encounter on that road.

I didn't think that I would have to fight people to let me try and help people. I didn't know that I was entering something that was not what it appeared to be. I want people to know this truth. People are addicted because people want them to be addicted. Their addiction is serving a purpose for someone else. The people claiming that they are involved in giving a shit about people with substance abuse problems don't give a shit about them. They have another motive and that is about themselves and has nothing to do with the people they claim they serve. They are like crows that descend on the bodies of the dead and then pick at their bones.

The government of this country benefits too much from addiction. It has no interest in helping those at the bottom of this sickness. They can easily be wiped off the table after they have lost their usefulness and become enough of a nuisance to be gotten rid of. The beauty of this design is they will sign up for their own demise, and it will look like an act of compassion; after all they were too broken to survive.

The people making decisions ask the most addicted people what they want and then follow their direction. If you ask an addicted person what they want, they will tell you they want you to give them drugs because they are addicted to drugs. Then you give them drugs; this makes no sense. We've already seen what they do with a safe supply; they sell it in order to buy street drugs. They don't want your safe supply to use it but only as a way to make money to buy what they really want. In both of Aaron Gun's Videos, "Vancouver is Dying" and "Canada is Dying" he identified where the safe supply going? To College and University Students. All the Harm Reductionists were doing was creating a new group of addicts. If that's what we want, then I guess that's what we will have.

I have felt some hope coming from Alberta's recent response to addiction. They have chosen to go the route of long-term treatment and have invested in a number of very large treatment centers. Alberta's Family Initiative were also the creators of the Brain Story, which sought to educate people on the effects of trauma on the brain and how to raise resilience in children. It seems that this province is much farther ahead in its approach to health and health education than the rest of Canada.

This is where we need to focus our attention. We need to help people get better. Addiction is damaging to people. It destroys their bodies and their brains. It is not a good long-term solution. This does not lead to any quality of life. People can and do recover. It makes absolutely no sense to just allow a significant group of people to choose to disable themselves through alcohol and drug use when this can be treated. Even if their choice had no repercussions for other people, it would still be something we should be motivated to treat because it is self-harming.

We need to help people realize that there is a reason to

get better. This is the pivotal piece I think people are missing. Everyone is caught up in the idea that people need to be able to make a choice when they are in no position to make a choice. They can't see a reason. Treatment requires that we help people find the desire to live again. We need to have humanity built into the treatment program to care enough for these people that we pull them back from the edge of that cliff and back into their lives. These are people who are killing themselves slowly but surely and in a horrible way. Do we have enough humanity to stop the horror, or are we just content to participate in this mass suicide and say we were just being kind?

Treatment requires getting people off the drugs they are using. It requires treating the physical body of the person, teaching and providing nutrition, helping the body to recover movement and strength, and addressing physical injuries or conditions. It requires treating the person's mental health because they may have disorders or illnesses that have never been addressed or ones they have just not been taking care of. This may include specific medication and/or therapy. They may need to learn how to live a healthier lifestyle and how to put a structure into their day. It is helpful to understand why drugs or alcohol were chosen as a coping mechanism and what problems came with that choice. Looking for alternate coping mechanisms is helpful. What were some of their life struggles that made drug use a necessity? Completing an ACE questionnaire would help in identifying the traumas they experienced and would point to some areas for trauma therapy. Identifying what skills they had, what their education was, and what they might need would allow them to become financially sustainable. They might need some occupational training.

There could be some value in creating businesses that could accommodate workplaces for people learning to adapt back into the normal world. They could learn skills and how to become part of the normal economy. In this stage, they could be living in some form of transitional housing until they are ready to transition out into regular living and find a job in the community. There could be some partnerships with local businesses if people were willing to buy into real solutions. This is not to say there would not be problems because this population is not the easiest to work with, and we have just spent many years training them in how to become completely nonfunctional.

I recently attended the Canadian Center on Substance Abuse's (CCSA) 2024 conference in Vancouver. I presented as a person of lived experience a creative piece involving 184 drawings set to music where I read three poems while this played behind me. One poem was about a mother who cannot grieve because no one wants to hear about her addicted daughter; one is my own story; and the last was the story of a thirteen-year-old child who loses her mother to alcoholism. The drawings were of addicted people, children and parents. It was the only presentation at the conference that showed the dark reality of addiction (this is Addiction https://youtu.be/2uLCPRr4BTU?si=I9oNFTH9HKjWZ-MF). The rest of the Conference was some pretense that everything in the world of substance use was just rosy.

I attended a presentation after presentation that failed to mention the reality of addiction. I was approached by a gentleman from Australia who said to me after one such presentation, "If I did what they are suggesting, all of my people would be dead." Later, I was seated on the plane beside one of the executives of the CCSA and he asked me what I thought of the conference. I said either you are lying, or you all drank the Kool-Aid. I explained that all they presented was this rosy picture of addiction, like using people were so nice. I said they obviously do not live in your neighborhood. He said he took offence because I didn't know where he lived. I asked him if women serviced their johns in his laneway, and he said no. I asked him if people fired guns in his backyard, and he said no. I asked if people yelled out, "I'll give you a blow job for twenty dollars on his street," and he said no. I said then they obviously don't live in your neighborhood. He wasn't very happy with our conversation, but I was tired of their lies.

The whole ugly story needs to be told. At the level of addiction, it is a different group of people that are caught. They did not just accidentally start using too much and it got out of hand. There's a whole lot of pain under that. That is what set the trap. That is what drives the insanity and the craziness.

Between who I was at the end of my using and who I am now is such a huge distance. Drugs and alcohol do not allow for developmental growth, emotional growth or moral growth. The longer you stay in that world the crazier it gets. If you are out on the street, then it can get really very sick because it's survival. The rules there are completely different than in the real world. If you are going to survive there, you are going to end up doing things you would never have considered before.

When you are addicted, you will have to deal with withdrawal because you will not always be able to get the drug you need. Withdrawal is painful, but it is not just because of the physical withdrawal itself, it is the constant pain you feel from just living. It becomes more acute when you are in withdrawal from the drugs. The drugs themselves no longer take it away, but without them it just feels worse. That's the trap; you have to keep using even though it no longer works, it just keeps the withdrawal at bay.

The only real way to fix it is to stop using and deal with the pain that lies underneath the addiction. That's the only way that has a chance of succeeding. That might require therapy and medication. There may be another path that will work, but addiction won't.

The reason why I wanted to write this book was to shine a light on madness. I entered into the world of addiction through my birth into an addicted family. It led me into my own addiction and my own becoming lost. I then entered into the world of what I thought was recovery from addiction, and that is where that madness really began to show itself. Where you take everything, you think makes sense and then do the opposite. Where the people with the least education appear to have more knowledge than the people at the top, and how can that be possible?

Here I refer to how many medical professionals thought that sending a seriously alcoholic person home with a prescription for benzodiazepines was an intelligent thing to do. Also, that we should leave an underage girl to visit the home of a pedophile nightly, while he sells her for crack or why the police are not all trained in human trafficking or why treatment tends to be a lottery.

But the biggest question I have is where we ever got the idea that people using drugs are nice people. That's the current mantra, and you can only say this if you don't live in the neighborhood where they live. It's absolutely infuriating if you do live in such a neighborhood because you will quickly see what happens to your rights, freedom and safety. If they decide to invalidate your rights, try and do something about it. They are very creative people when it comes to retaliation. They will quickly make you sorry if you ask them to stop doing something they don't wish to stop. You can call the police, but that could result in much more serious retaliation. Before you take these guys on, be sure you are ready for the game. It's not going to be a simple situation. As I referred to my neighbor who got three slashed tires, her car keyed, and her windshield smashed for asking the neighbors to stop sending their dog over to our place to do his business. Without proof there is nothing she can do but pay for the damage they caused her and install cameras where she parks her car. But the government feels they have a right to use their drugs because, after all, people who use substances are nice people.

How in the hell did we turn the world so upside down? I was an addict and nothing about that was positive. I was not my best self. I was completely lost and going absolutely nowhere. I would never want to be that person again. I was not capable of anything that could be called productive. No matter how much I wanted to be a good person I was incapable of being that. My addiction owned me. It drove me into darker and darker places in my mind.

There were so many times I felt like I was losing my mind. I could not stop using drugs even though I was not getting anything positive from them anymore. I became hopelessly suicidal in the end. I never have a desire to go back because I remember how terrible it was at the end, and I never want to be there again. Being trapped in the need to use drugs to avoid withdrawal, knowing it will not really help the way you feel about your life, is a horrible place to find yourself.

The problem with addiction is that it is complicated by the fact that it not only hurts the person who is struggling with it, but it hurts so many others as well. A person can have heart disease, and they don't end up beating their children to death or stealing everything they can get their hands on. The behaviors that surround the use of drugs and alcohol are often appalling. The idea that if we just give them the drugs and that will be the answer is ridiculous because intoxicated people do not behave well. We can give them an injection site and a disposable box for their needles, and yet they will still dump them wherever. Drunk people will not behave quietly. People on methamphetamine are not safe parents, and we know that people who are addicted exchange their safe supply for street drugs and that safe supply is sold to college and university students.

Addiction requires an active program of recovery and treatment. If it caused no harm, then we could say that people have a right to make their own choices, but addiction by its nature is not a choice, and by its nature it harms everything around it. It is worse than a contagious disease; it is a toxic disease. Those who benefit from it are predators. The reason for addiction is trauma, and addiction is not a treatment for trauma but an opportunity to cause more trauma. Addiction is the way we throw away people that we choose not to protect. It's the way we disempower them. Lost in their addiction they will never know what their own truth really is. Addiction makes money, and recovery threatens that.

It's important that people see the current trend for what it is. The Government is dealing addiction. I believe that it is also flirting with another disturbing idea. It is currently on hold, but if the Government gets its way, it will find a way to offer MAID to those addicted to drugs. This will be its "final solution" for addiction, a way to clear problems like the tent cities of Vancouver. I left the addiction field when I realized that I could no longer, in good faith, be part of what was happening.

I have thirty-two years clean and sober. I still attend twelve-step meetings. I still reach out to others. This is my last goodbye to the addiction field. I never planned on leaving quietly. I've intentionally not named anyone because there is no need. The problems were across the board, and I'm sure they were similar across the country. If you recognize yourself here, maybe you might think about those who suffered rather than your own egos because we've all seen enough of your egos to last a lifetime. To all those who died, I am so very sorry that I was unable to stop those in power from throwing you away. To your family members, I am also so sorry that you lost your family members in such a cruel and callous way. I hope by telling some of your stories that I will have rectified my own inability to have been able to stop what was going on. I will never forget any of you; I still see your faces in my mind.

I have come to believe that I suffered a moral injury from my work in the addiction field. I saw so much wrong that I was unable to do anything about, regardless of what I tried to do. This industry showed me what it was capable of, and I was not immune to its threats or attacks. I went through a lot personally. I had people who were in positions of power over me who lied about me, who denied me my basic rights and who made me realize how unhealthy this field was.

In one job, I was personally harassed in my workplace and denied time off while others around me were not. I had a manager question my mental health in such a derogatory way as it was insulting. It was during COVID and we were talking as a group about how COVID was affecting us. I was living alone at the time, and I commented that I had tried to join a discussion group online to help with the isolation. It was on black issues which had always interested me, but I found out you had to be black to join the group and I mentioned I was disappointed. My manager called me aside later and was concerned I was psychotic because I thought I was black. I was so taken aback that I thought she had lost it. She knew I had a mental health diagnosis and all I could think of was that she really needed to get some mental health training because what she had just done was completely ridiculous and extremely offensive.

I did need to see a counselor when I was receiving physiotherapy for a car accident where I was hit by a car as a pedestrian, but I was denied the opportunity to take time off. I worked for weeks with only one colleague because one or the other was away, and there were a number of days I worked alone with a full load of clients present in the program. I was the most recent hirer into this program while my colleagues had both been working in this program for over ten years. Despite this, I was denied time off.

I was told that, in one instance, I didn't give them enough notice. I was asking for an afternoon off where there would be no clients scheduled unless you had booked them yourself. I had called my manager since I was away on an arranged activity where my salary was being paid for by someone other than my workplace with my workplace's permission. She agreed to give me the time off since there was no issue it would cause for the other staff members. The supervisor above her said I couldn't have the time off because I hadn't given enough notice. It was Friday and I was asking for the following Thursday afternoon off. I asked how much notice I needed to give, and he said he couldn't give me an answer. I asked him if I could leave early because I was scheduled to take a plane to Toronto. He refused even though there would be absolutely nothing I would be doing at the workplace that afternoon. I had no behavioral issues in my work and was a good employee. There was just no reason to do what he did other than he could do that. I was exhausted from working constantly with only one other staff member and, at times, working alone with a full load of clients and never getting a break.

I had been going to physical therapy early in the morning because I had been in a car accident where I was hit as a pedestrian walking across the street on the way to work one morning. This had caused a knee injury and an injury to my buttocks. It had killed an area of nerves in my buttocks, and I was having a number of different treatments to see if they could reduce the size of the dead part. This began causing me to have traumatic nightmares from the incident where I had been attacked by my manager at the bank. I never saw that coming, so my sleep was being affected which wasn't being helped by the high stress of being unsupported and overworked. This was the reason I had decided to see a counselor, and I had to stop physiotherapy. I had been accused of not informing them of the counseling appointment even though the appointment took place when I was being paid by someone other than them, and I had asked these people for permission. It was also at the very end of the day. I finally just called my doctor and asked her to book me off on stress leave because I couldn't handle the harassment anymore. This was an agency that helps people. I found out they were quite capable of hurting people.

When I finally walked away from it completely, I realized I had no other choice. It took some time to recover from what had happened to me personally, but I always knew I would write this book. I realized that someone needed to tell this story for the sake of all the people who had been harmed by the decisions of others and the very unhealthy people who head this field. I was nearly another casualty of this world. Trying to fight against what was going on was never received well. At some point, I had to realize I didn't have the power to fight it.

What I could do is tell people about it. I could tell other people's truths because so many of them would never get that chance. I know if they or their family members pick up this book, they will know who their people are. I cared very deeply for you. There were many times I cried because I could not save your loved ones or get them the help they most certainly deserved. I want you to know that I will never forget you. You kept whispering in my ear, please tell the truth about this. To those who made it out, God bless you. This is my story as well as yours, because I walked in the same world as you. We can do so much better than we have done so far. To the treatment providers, those struggling with addiction deserve so much more than the ugly life they currently live in. They cannot see clearly but you can. For God's sake lift them up. Don't leave them in a living hell. That's a harder road, and it requires a bit more effort, but these people are worth it.

***

I have been a poet for most of my life. I have tried many times to write about my experience with addiction in poetry. This is one of those attempts:

The Cost

I paid the cost right from the start and I paid it year to year.
So easily discarded in the bottom of my mother's glass of beer
The last child born into a marriage forever doomed to fail.
When my father ran to escape prison, I faced a different kind of jail.
The seeringness of her bitterness like a magnifying glass placed over me.
The last thing that she needed was all that she could see.
Just an act of fate and nothing that I'd really ever done.
A twisted game of chance and this was all that I had won.
One more mouth to feed she didn't need is what she often said.
And when I turned nineteen is when she hoped that she'd be dead
The things my siblings never heard were what I heard too many times to bear.
How many times I sat on the front stairs of our place with that silent far away stare.
No chance to be a child, only to prove that I had a right to be.
She told me I was never wanted and there in lied the cost demanded of me.
I somehow owed her for being the extra burden on her plate.
And there were times I could see where her anger rose to hate.
Like somehow, I represented everything that had gone wrong within her life.
Like all the dark clouds had come in the day they cut the umbilical cord with the knife

And I could feel the darkness when she looked into my eyes.
And it never really mattered that her projection had been lies.
Because as a child I had no way to defend myself from her abuse
So, in the end I would just become the child that she would use.
Trying to prove I was worth something by giving up my right to be a child.
Willing to do anything she wanted like a number that was dialed.
Until my own identity was gone, and my feelings became hers
But still unable to escape her rages or being the subject of her slurs.
All the while my siblings came and went about their lives as children do.
While I was chained in shame and guilt by my mother's point of view
Never good enough to rise above the crime that I committed.
Of being born when all was lost when I should not have been admitted
It was like my admission changed the play from a romance to a tragedy.
Like I'd taken everything that was perfect and stole away its majesty
But I hadn't planned my birth, two people performed the act of my creation.
And the burden placed upon my shoulders left me with chronic suicidal ideation.
The child of their neglect, born into a broken home
I would spend most of my life in the pain of being left alone.
Unable to wash away the stain of the mistakes my parents made.
The words my mother spoke tattooed on my brain would never fade.
The effect was to leave me broken until there was something wrong with me.
When you grow inside the darkness then it's only darkness that you see
So. when she invited me into her addiction I eventually agreed.
And it wasn't like I hadn't seen where that ugly path would lead.
But I had nothing to lose at that point because I'd already lost.
I'd spent my entire life in pain, so I'd already paid the cost.
Why not plummet to the bottom it wasn't very far to fall.
Afterall I was suicidal so why not lose it all?.
And at first it numbed my mind and kept some of the pain away
But all it really did was save it for another rainy day.
And just as she predicted she died just before I turned nineteen.

Leaving her youngest child's mind so twisted with all that was unseen.
Carrying a baggage of shame and guilt into another relationship doomed to fail.
Into another half a lifetime of neglect and another lonely jail
Writing the ugly messages deeper into my already damaged brain
Like I'd spent far too long soaking in a bath of acid rain
Adding drugs of various kinds in a search to obliterate my mind
I tried so hard to escape reality, but escape was hard to find.
Reality kept returning with another batch of shame.
As the pages of my wrongs kept turning in another drunken game
Caught inside a trap I'd somehow set up on my own.
The day I took the first drug it was my life I would disown.
Walking into walls as I turned myself round and round.
The fact that I was lost was all that I had found.
An adult with a child inside that had never been a child.
With an uncanny ability to remember so nothing could be filed
Stuck in a place in time that replicated too much of the past.
Playing Russian Roulette with drug use in a hope that I wouldn't last.
With my mental health teetering on the brink of the edge of a cliff
Sitting against a wall with an AK47 while I smoked another spliff.
Contemplating a violent end where more than I would pay the price.
The grandiosity of the image and my anger creating the fuel to entice
All the while seeking another exit and hoping I could find another door.
A part of me knowing this was not what my life was meant for.
And finally, the door opened, and I slipped in through the gate.
And closed the door behind me and hoped to erase my ugly fate.
But I could not close the door on all that happened as it raged on through my mind.
Memories of a lifetime living in the world of the unkind
All that was said and done had marked me deep into my soul.
And I might have reached for recovery but for the longest time self-destruction had been my only goal.
I had hated myself for so long I couldn't bear to see my own reflection.
And if there was a self-inside it could barely reach detection

There was a rage that simmered deep threatening to swallow all of me.
There was a depression that was so dark at times I could barely see.
Moods that rose and fell without warning leaving me confused and so unsure.
Too many sleepless nights fearing I couldn't possibly have a future.
Medications for a mental illness that I had to accept that I now had.
With suicidal ideation raging through the days and nights also driving me mad
So many times, I wasn't sure I'd make it fighting the war inside of me.
I thought that I'd already paid the cost, but I still had to pay another fee.
The fee for all the mistakes I made while I ran away inside my addiction.
All of those I hurt so casually while I thrashed out blindly in my affliction.
All the things I said that I couldn't remember but my anxiety made it clear.
The pain reflected in another's face revealed my actions as if they were a mirror.
Nothing like coming face to face with yourself guilty of all that was done to you.
Wondering how you can live with yourself or ever have a different point of view.
Wondering why you shouldn't just end it all rather than continue with the pain.
Unable to see the possibility of ever washing away an iota of the stain.
Years of darkness mediated by the rooms where others shared.
And slowly over time I came to realize there were others that now cared.
Bit by bit the painful changes happened, and humanity returned.
So much I had never experienced before so I couldn't say that they were things that I relearned.
I was in a different world from the one I left behind.
Trying to find my bearings and trying to heal my mind
Trying for the first time to decide who I really was
After years as a puppet where addiction decides what it does
Still an observer from my childhood I watched my own journey to be free.
All the twists and turns, the therapies and everything else that I could see.
To try to understand the path I took, how I came to be so lost.

Never wanting to repeat the mistakes I made or ever again to pay the cost.
Somehow, I got invited to try and help others make it to the other side.
I knew the price that could be paid because I had almost died.
The invitation appealed to the place where I had once been lost.
The place where I had given up my childhood as the final cost.
But I thought I could make a difference and do something that was worth doing.
Help others find a way out of the darkness of addiction into a life that was worth viewing.
I was smart enough to go to university and get an education.
And I took the relevant courses and exams to get the designation.
But what I had lived was the greatest asset because I knew it from the heart.
I knew what addiction does and how it tears your life apart.
I'd seen it from all sides, so I knew it face to face.
It's something you can't learn in school because it comes from a very different place.
It's how I knew each person seeking help because I'd been right where they stood.
I knew the cost they paid in their addiction, and I knew how much more it could.
But what I didn't see until later were the people that ran the addiction field
It wasn't until twenty-seven years later that I realized that it was my fate that had been sealed.
Over and over, I found myself in the dysfunction I tried so hard to leave behind.
The tangled web of agencies so focused on themselves they left their clients in a bind.
Decisions made that made no sense except to make a power play.
The lives lost in the balance to give someone the last say.
Those that died unseen because their lives were never seen as having meaning.
Policies that claimed compassion while their actions were really, just demeaning.

And if you fought for the life of your client, you only sealed their fate.
As they closed the door even tighter, and you became the one they'd hate.
Agencies in a pissing match on who had the last word on your client.
And when their actions led to a death, they were suddenly very silent.
Hospitals that threw your client out into the street
Claiming they weren't worth helping because they were the author of their own defeat.
Until finally addiction was a good thing, and they should just be allowed to use.
And they'd even give them the drugs, so they'd have nothing left to lose.
And that's when I finally walked away because I felt like I was lost.
Like all those years ago when I had paid the cost
Only now the loss was greater because I couldn't see the hope.
It was all a game of chance and the ability to cope.
When I entered into recovery, I thought I crossed to the other side.
I thought when I left the world of active addiction, I left the world where people lied.
It was a rather naïve belief because it really wasn't any different here.
Except I was no longer using, and I was no longer filled with fear.
But the ugly just continued on, people hurting people because they could.
And I wondered why I thought I could ever find a world that could be good.
I found myself alone again discarded by my kin.
And realized there hadn't been much of my life where I hadn't been broken.
And now I live a lot in silence, the place for those alone
I still give my time to others; I sometimes talk to others on the phone.
I have a few friends and sometimes they find the time to spend with me.
I try to spend some time in nature because that's the kindest place to be.
I seek spirituality hoping I can find a way to understand.
I've gone to the ancestral home of my people to connect to my motherland.
The closest I came to true connection was with a bunny I recently lost.
I loved him with all of my heart but then he died and once more I paid the cost.

It's really hard to comment on the place I find myself in
It has been a long and difficult life in the places where I've been.
There have been moments of magic that told me that there was something that was there?
Woven through the places where I saw so much despair.
There were many faces along the way where I hoped I helped others make it.
But it was often so very difficult because you'd think you'd see safety but mistake it.
Too many wolves in sheep's clothing hiding among the places where people reached out a hand.
And I saw far too many needlessly fall for nothing and for what I'll never understand.
The trauma left its mark, there was a broken part of me.
I knew what beauty there could be, but the trauma charged a fee.
There was a deep dark sadness that often came silently in like an ocean wave.
And it took everything that I could muster to find some of me to save.
So today I live a survival game, and I never know if I will win.
Somedays I can see a lot of light and other days the light grows dim.
I'd like to think I stood for what was right but there are people who tore me down.
And given all the pain of my childhood it's been hard to hold my ground.
The child whose mother told her she wasn't wanted still struggles to find her worth
She still hears the echo in her mind asking, why were you ever given birth?
And even though I understand it was a mother's desperation and not me.
All the years she said it to me was a pain that wouldn't let me be.
It left me standing on uncertain ground unsteady on my feet.
That much more in danger to suffer just one more defeat.
And in a world where throwing stones is such a natural game to play
I wore a lot of bruises for the truths I tried to say.
I'd like to believe I've lived my life as honestly as I could.
But I know in life there have been few people who have ever understood.

And really why would they, life is hard enough to live.
To expect someone to understand, is to expect more than they can give.
After all, we live in a world where most of us are lost.
And in the end, there must be those who are left to pay the cost.

Acknowledgements

I would like to acknowledge some great men who shone a light into a very dark place where a young, rejected child lived for the most part alone inside herself. I found hope in the courage and strength of people such as Martin Luther King, Malcom X, Eldridge Cleaver, Stephen Biko, Nelson Mandela, and Gandhi. Without their light I wouldn't have been able to stand alone for most of my childhood and have survived.

Although my mother was unwell and impacted by her own life experiences, the tragedy of her life taught me what not to do at the turning point in my life. I have always loved her, and I always will. She left me with a lifetime of emotional damage, but she was very damaged herself.

It is hard when I look at my road through the world of addiction recovery and the addiction field itself to say something here. There was so much unhealthiness in this world. There were those who were helpful to me in my own journey—Rita Hughes, Pauline Kelly-Smith, Monica Forst, to name a few. The 12-step community was very helpful and still is a part of my life. They became my family for the most part.

There are a number of people from recovery that have become good friends and that I am very grateful for their presence in my life. They are MJ, Karen M., Karen L., Debbie M., April L., Rob M., Dan, Ygal, Steve, Julie, JB, Mike, and many more.

I learned a lot from some important people like Terence Gorski, whose work on Relapse Prevention was so instrumental in helping people who many just thought could not achieve recovery.

Vincent J Felitti, whose work on the Adverse Childhood

Events study opened up so much thought on the role of trauma in addiction and was such an important part of my learning.

I was extremely proud when the Alberta Family Initiative took that study and created the Brain Story which was a 19-module free online course that educated anyone who wanted to make use of it on how significant this study was and how children were affected and then how we could combat this by building stronger brains through encouraging resilience in children. I had the unique opportunity to be one of the people who got to be involved in creating a project to encourage others to access this course and raise awareness about this course and their resources.

I also would like to thank SAMHSA for all the work that they do and all of the great publications they make available. I was always looking for information to help with clients and this was always an amazing resource.

One report that I found particularly helpful was the American Surgeon General's report called Finding Addiction in America 2016 which presented one of the best neurological explanations of addiction. When working in this field you were always confronted with trying to provide the legitimacy of addiction as a real medical issue with symptoms and a progression. This report adequately laid this out. I did a presentation on this showing how the neuroscience also mirrored the lived experience.

I'd also like to thank Aaron Gunn for his tireless reporting on the addiction story in Canada. He produced three films, "Vancouver is Dying" (https://youtu.be/PT8OU8Yhs_s?si=QZsbNj6tZIMd8NV_), "Canada is Dying" (https://youtu.be/_RaWzJUeT0o?si=3wziOUTsIyLFw5kN), and "The Deadliest Scandal in Canadian History" (https://youtu.be/aoBEyJu3ctA?si=nW5XvCaNBY9xDI0z). His work was absolutely stellar in telling what was going on behind the scenes of Canada's safe supply which ended up diverting close to 100% of Dilaudid into organized crime across Canada. These pills were then sold at $2.00 a pill on Canadian streets to novel users creating a whole new population of opiate users. This was happening while lead figures in Providence Health Care and the BC Centre on Substance Use all decided to buy heroin companies. Thank you, Aaron, for being on the ground and finding the truth. Check out his videos to get the complete picture.

Dr. Bruce Perry has been a constant inspiration for me as a mentor. This a man I see as a great humanitarian and a man who demonstrates for me how we need to be in relation to each other. He is a neuroscientist and a child psychiatrist, and I found his work early on in my career. I have read many of his research articles, I have seen him numerous times in person and read his books, *The Boy Who was Raised as a Dog*, *Born for Love and What Happened to You.* I kept a picture I managed to get of him and myself at my work on the wall to remind me of the importance of being a caring human being.

Gabor Mate is a Canadian doctor who has done so much amazing work not only in addiction but in trauma but again in understanding human struggle and the need for healing. I have met and talked to him and read many of his books including *In the Realm of the Hungry Ghosts*, *Scattered Minds*, *When the Body says No*, and *The Myth of Normal.* He has spoken all over the world and is a wise man with much to teach us all.

Lastly I'd like to thank Jordan Peterson. I have followed Dr. Peterson's lectures and talks for quite a number of years now. For a while I was unaware of the controversy surrounding him because I was only listening to his talks and not the debates and arguments that were occurring on YouTube. What I have found is that his talks have been very helpful for me. Often when I feel lost, or I feel like I just have had enough, I search out one of his talks and I find a lot of benefit from this. I live alone and so I don't have the benefit of someone I can talk to when things are tough or something difficult has happened. I have to manage these things on my own. A while back I developed a routine response to difficult times where I look to people who I know are smarter than I am and who have a lot of intelligent and sensitive things to say, and I listen to them at those times. Jordan Peterson is one of those people. There are few others like Carl Jung and Maya Angelou who, although not alive, have many examples of their wisdom on YouTube. I think I learned this as a young child, and it still works for me. There is so much wisdom out there and the internet makes it easy to find.

About Atmosphere Press

Founded in 2015, Atmosphere Press was built on the principles of Honesty, Transparency, Professionalism, Kindness, and Making Your Book Awesome. As an ethical and author-friendly hybrid press, we stay true to that founding mission today.

If you're a reader, enter our giveaway for a free book here:

SCAN TO ENTER
BOOK GIVEAWAY

If you're a writer, submit your manuscript for consideration here:

SCAN TO SUBMIT
MANUSCRIPT

And always feel free to visit Atmosphere Press and our authors online at atmospherepress.com. See you there soon!

About the Author

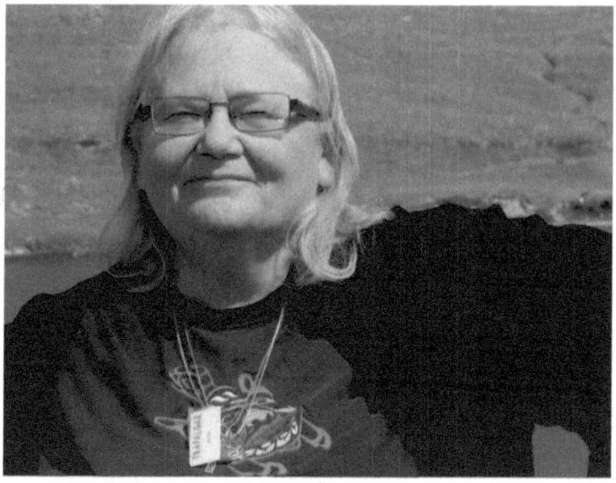

Karen James spent 27 years working in the field of addiction treatment and counseling with a wide range of clients from teens to those in conflict with the law in Canada. She was a creative child who grew up in a family impacted by addiction and as a result of that impact she became addicted too. After the loss of that family and recovery she worked to help others. She is both an artist and a poet and has tried to champion the rights of those who have no voices. This book is an attempt to right some of those wrongs but also encourage some accountability in recovery.

www.ingramcontent.com/pod-product-compliance
Lightning Source LLC
LaVergne TN
LVHW100302210926
848480LV00003B/1003